Atlas of Reconstructive Burn Surgery

Roger E. Salisbury, M.D.

Associate Professor of Surgery
Division of Plastic and Reconstructive Surgery and Surgery of the Hand
Director, North Carolina Jaycee Burn Center
Department of Surgery
University of North Carolina at Chapel Hill
Chapel Hill, North Carolina

A. Griswold Bevin, M.D.

Professor of Surgery
Chief, Division of Plastic and Reconstructive Surgery and Surgery of the Hand
Department of Surgery
University of North Carolina at Chapel Hill
Chapel Hill, North Carolina

with a contribution by

Freddi S. Salisbury

Cosmetologist
North Carolina Jaycee Burn Center
Chapel Hill, North Carolina

and illustrations by

Harold A. Rydberg, Medical Illustrator

Department of Medical Illustration and Photography
University of North Carolina at Chapel Hill
Chapel Hill, North Carolina

1981

W. B. SAUNDERS COMPANY   Philadelphia   London   Toronto   Sydney

W. B. Saunders Company: West Washington Square
Philadelphia, PA 19105

1 St. Anne's Road
Eastbourne, East Sussex BN21 3UN, England

1 Goldthorne Avenue
Toronto, Ontario M8Z 5T9, Canada

9 Waltham Street
Artarmon, N.S.W. 2064, Australia

Library of Congress Cataloging in Publication Data

Salisbury, Roger E

Atlas of reconstructive burn surgery.

1. Burns and scalds—Surgery. 2. Surgery, Plastic.
I. Bevin, A. Griswold, joint author. II. Title.
III. Title: Reconstructive burn surgery. [DNLM: 1. Burns—
Surgery—Atlases. 2. Surgery, Plastic—Atlases.
WO 517 S167a]

RD96.4.S23   617'.110592   80-25571

ISBN 0-7216-7903-X

Atlas of Reconstructive Burn Surgery   ISBN 0-7216-7903-X

© 1981 by W. B. Saunders Company. Copyright under the Uniform Copyright Convention. Simultaneously published in Canada. All rights reserved. This book is protected by copyright. No part of it may be reproduced, stored in a retrieval system, or transmitted in any form or by any means, electronic, mechanical, photocopying, recording, or otherwise, without written permission from the publisher. Made in the United States of America. Press of W. B. Saunders Company. Library of Congress catalog card number 80-25571.

Last digit is the print number: 9 8 7 6 5 4 3 2 1

*This work is dedicated to those
remarkable people who have suffered
the agony of agonies.
It is our hope that it will stimulate
and assist others in offering their
talents and skill to these patients.*

Preface

The burn team taking the responsibility for reconstructing and rehabilitating the thermally injured patient is working under a time constraint that is not always appreciated. Vocational rehabilitation counselors have learned that, if the patient is not returned to work within 18 months following acute injury, the chances of meaningful re-employment decrease geometrically with time. Thus, a particular operation may be a technical success for the surgeon, but may have no meaning in the patient's future.

A rehabilitation plan must be designed for the patient, with timely surgery as only one part of the plan. Each patient is evaluated by the entire burn team, including occupational and physical therapist, nurse, vocational rehabilitation counselor, social worker, chaplain, play therapist, psychiatrists, and surgeons. Family problems and nonmedical considerations that might hinder progress are explored. The patient's medical situation and functional prognosis are discussed with his employer, to involve him in the rehabilitation program. The importance of this step cannot be overemphasized because, in today's job market, the employer can always find an unburned candidate to replace your patient.

To facilitate return to work, all surgery is categorized as either essential or desirable. Essential surgery is defined as that necessary to allow independent function for daily living or to make possible the patient's re-employment. Desirable surgery is that which makes the patient look better, and restores anatomical integrity. Essential surgery is performed first to return the patient to work. Desirable surgery is then performed periodically throughout a variable period after re-employment.

The reconstructive surgery described on the following pages is intended to be a guide, not an encyclopedia. Thus, no attempt is made to document every procedure for a given deformity. We have organized the book anatomically, and have dealt with the most commonly seen problems for each area.

In the realization that burn facilities differ not only in size but in the types of surgeons working in them, the procedures chosen are those that might have appeal to general, orthopedic, otolaryngologic, and plastic surgeons. The esoteric operation or the technical maneuver that is being done only at one institution in the U.S. is intentionally avoided. Our purpose is to describe a philosophy of surgical care for the reader who may not see burned patients frequently, as well as for the specialist. Thus, we have selected operative procedures that we personally have found to be safe and to have a good chance for success. We have stressed basic wound management techniques and basic surgical principles.

A.G.B.

R.E.S.

Contents

Part 1 Head, Face, and Neck

Burns of the Scalp and Skull 3

1	Burn Alopecia	4
2	Scalp Rotation Flaps	8
3	Visor Scalp Flap for Restoration of Anterior Hairline	14
4	Loss of the Scalp and Destruction of the Underlying Pericranium	18
5	Loss of the Scalp and Underlying Skull: Decortication	22

Reconstruction of the Thermally Injured Ear 25

6	Reconstruction of the Superior Helix by Retroauricular Skin Advancement	26
7	Cartilage Defect of the Superior Helix	28
8	The Contracted Ear Lobule	30

Burns of the Face 33

9	Anatomical Imperatives and Esthetic Facial Units: The Art of Seeing	34
10	The Eyebrow: Total and Partial Loss	40
11	Upper Eyelid Ectropion	46
12	Lower Eyelid Ectropion	50
13	Resurfacing the Nose	52
14	Radiation Injury of the Lip	55
15	Reconstruction of the Oral Commissures	58
16	Perioral Hypertrophic Burn Scars: Upper Lip and Lower Lip-Chin Unit	66
17	Reconstruction of the Lower Labial Sulcus	70
18	The Everted Lower Lip	76
19	Lower Lip-Chin Esthetic Facial Unit	80
20	Re-creation of the Anatomical Angles of the Lower Facial Unit	84

Burn Contractures of the Neck 89

21	Cervical Contracture At or Above the Level of the Hyoid	90
22	Cervical Contracture or Scarring Involving the Entire Anterior Surface of the Neck	95
23	Cervical Contracture Below the Level of the Hyoid	102

CONTENTS

Part 2 Upper Extremity

24	The Axilla	108
25	Management of Elbow Contractures	112
26	Peripheral Nerve Loss Secondary to Electrical Injury	116
27	Heterotopic Ossification: Radioulnar Synostosis	126
28	Dorsal and Volar Wrist Contractures: Abduction of the Thumb	132
29	The Metacarpal Hand: An Opposable Cleft	138
30	The Accessory Hand: Selective Amputation	140
31	Excision and Grafting of the Dorsum of the Hand	144
32	Palm and Finger Contractures	150
33	Metacarpophalangeal Capsulotomy and Proximal Interphalangeal Arthrodesis	156
34	Boutonnière Deformity	164
35	Adduction Contracture of the Thumb	168
36	Scarring of Dorsal Thumb Web Skin: Anatomical Considerations	172
37	Pollicization	174
38	Burn Syndactyly: The "Hourglass" Procedure	180
39	Dorsal Adduction Contractures of the Fingers	186
40	Abduction Contracture of the Small Finger	190

Part 3 Trunk, Genitalia, and Lower Extremity

41	Caudal Contracture of the Breast	196
42	Lateral Contracture of the Breast	202
43	Loss of Breast Volume and Destruction of the Nipple-Areola Complex	206
44	Reconstruction of the Nipple-Areola Complex	212
45	Breast Reconstruction Using the Latissimus Dorsi Myocutaneous Flap	216
46	Burns of the Genitalia	222
47	Reconstruction of the Groin: The Tensor Fasciae Latae Myocutaneous Flap	228
48	Contractures of the Knee	232
49	Knee: The Lateral Gastrocnemius Myocutaneous Flap	236
50	Knee: The Medial Gastrocnemius Myocutaneous Flap	242
51	Coverage Near the Knee: The Sartorius Muscle Flap	246
52	Foot: Plantar Surface Injury	250
53	Dorsal Foot Contracture with Deformity of the Toes	254

Part 4 Cosmetics: A Nonsurgical Alternative

54	Cosmetics: A Nonsurgical Alternative	260
	Index	265

Head, Face, and Neck

Burns of the Scalp and Skull

The late problems resulting from burns of the scalp and skull will vary with the area and depth of the initial injury. These may be grouped in the following way:

a. Burn alopecia, or patchy areas of hairless scalp with intervening areas of hair growth.

b. Loss of the anterior hairline owing to hairless scalp that is present anteriorly and backward toward the vertex.

c. Loss of the scalp and destruction of the underlying pericranium.

d. Loss of the scalp and destruction of the underlying skull.

In the individual patient there may be several different levels of injury, and generally the deepest involvement will dictate the necessary type of reconstruction. The physiology of healing of the scalp and skull is complex. Early management of burn injuries with respect to preservation of the galea, the periosteum, and the skull itself will often determine the need for late reconstructive procedures. In most cases a reasonably functional and esthetic result can be achieved with a combination of aggressive early treatment, later surgical reconstruction, and modalities such as cosmetics and hair pieces.

1

Burn Alopecia

The Problem

When patchy, full-thickness burns of the scalp leave several areas of alopecia, it may not be possible to camouflage them even if the remaining hair is allowed to grow long. Often, these problems occur in children to whom a full hair piece to cover the defects is not readily acceptable. The ideal patient is one who has areas of alopecia not exceeding 20 to 30 per cent of the scalp surface, with relatively normal hair growth in the intervening regions. Serial excision of these areas may be performed over a period of time, resulting in an improved appearance.

Technique

Although the mechanism(s) for successful results (using serial excision of areas of alopecia, narrowing them to acceptable size) are unclear, several concepts have been proposed. One is simply that, with excised wounds closed under some tension, the remodeling that occurs actually attenuates the surrounding scalp and causes a certain amount of "spreading" of the distance between existing hair follicles. Another concept is that of "intussusceptive growth" of hair follicles in areas that have been approximated. Finally, it has been suggested that there is an enhancement of hair follicle function and perhaps even a form of hyperplasia in scalp that has been undermined, causing a type of "delay," with increased circulation as is seen with the circulatory physiology in delayed pedicle flaps in various other regions of the body.

From a practical point of view, however, it is possible to excise the areas of the bald scalp serially in as many as five or six procedures for an individual area, so that the resulting scar is narrow enough to be covered with hair that does not have to be unusually long.

Figure 1–1. This young patient has several areas of burn alopecia. A small anterior tuft of hair is present near the forehead, and a midline strip of hair over the vertex. There are additional small areas of alopecia in the temporal regions.

Figure 1–2. The right side of this patient's scalp is shown, with areas of alopecia.

Figure 1–3. The initial excision of an area of alopecia is seen. The first incision is planned for the geographical center of the particular area. The surrounding bald scalp is undermined at the level of the periosteum of the skull to achieve as much mobility as possible. Ellipsoidal excision of from one-fifth to one-third of the original area is carried out.

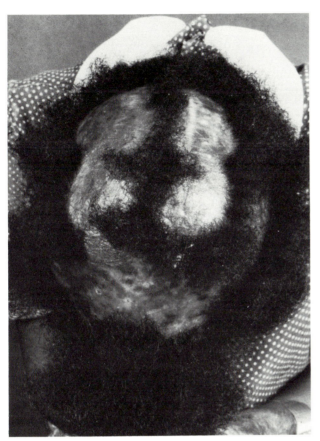

Figure 1-1

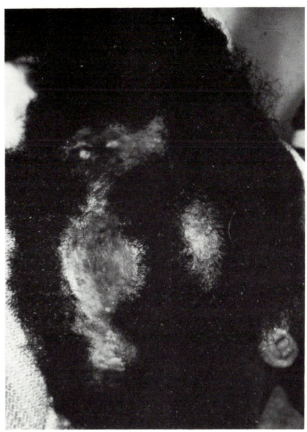

Figure 1-2

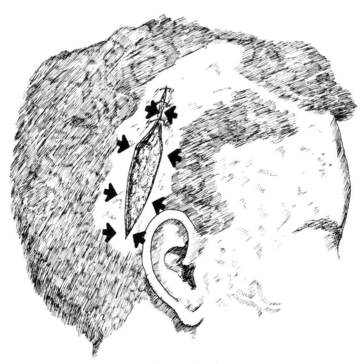

Figure 1-3

Figure 1-4. Horizontal mattress sutures of 4-0 monofilament material are used to insure edge-to-edge approximation of the wound, and these are often tied under modest tension. The sutures are placed approximately 1 cm apart to distribute tension reasonably, and if there is gaping of the wound between these sutures, several fine 5-0 interrupted sutures are placed for final approximation. Other areas seen in Figure 1-1 have been treated simultaneously.

Figure 1-5. The patient is shown after the right supra-auricular area has been excised, in addition to the previously noted areas.

Figures 1-6, 1-7. After final excision at several surgical procedures of all the areas initially present, the patient's hair has grown out approximately 1 or 2 inches in most areas, and is now sufficient to camouflage the resulting narrow operative scars.

Pitfalls and Solutions

1. Patients must be selected carefully so that those with excessively large areas of alopecia are not submitted to repeated operations that do not result in easily covered scars. Such individuals must be treated with other surgical maneuvers, or fitted with hair pieces.

2. Areas of alopecia that are contiguous with normal, hairless skin of the face or neck must not be treated by serial excision. Muscular forces in these areas will actually widen the scars toward the facial or neck regions. Only areas of alopecia within the hair-bearing confines of the scalp are acceptable for serial excision.

3. The hair must not be shaved closely prior to surgery. If remaining hair adjacent to areas of alopecia is sparse, close shaving may obliterate the margins. The hair should be cut to a length of one-eighth to one-fourth of an inch so that landmarks are preserved.

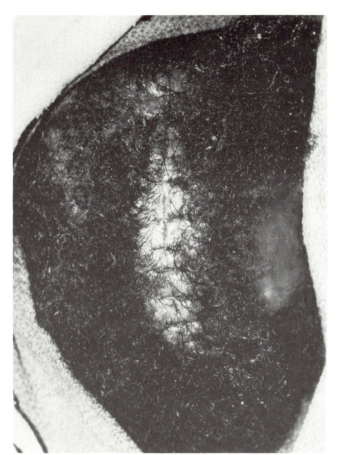

Figure 1-4

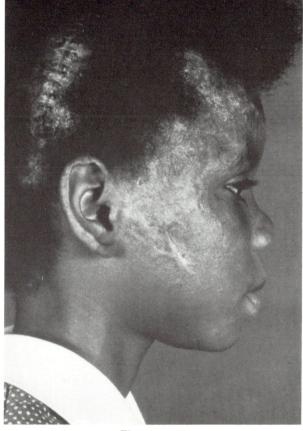

Figure 1-5

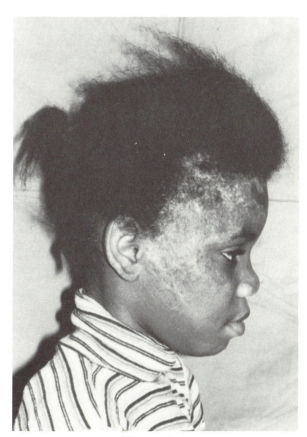

Figure 1-6

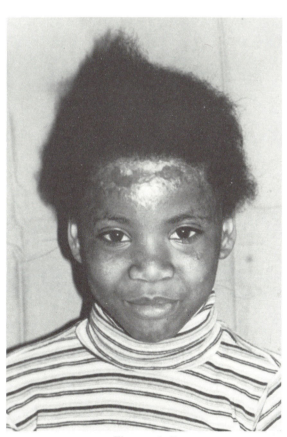

Figure 1-7

2

Scalp Rotation Flaps

The Problem

In the normal, intact state the entire scalp is actually a large pedicle. The blood supply to the scalp is derived entirely from the paired superficial temporal arteries and their branches, and from the paired occipital arteries. Usually, some additional blood supply occurs through the distal extensions of the supraorbital vessels. No significant blood supply enters from the underlying galea, periosteum, or skull. The scalp can thus be divided into areas from which pedicle flaps, based on one or more of the constant vascular pedicles, can be elevated and transposed to other locations. These flaps may be bi- or unipedicled.

Technique

Figure 2–1. Several sites for developing scalp pedicle flaps are illustrated. The paired superficial temporal and occipital arteries and their branches provide the vascular basis for these flaps. Flaps based on the superficial temporal arterial system can extend to the midline of the skull, and have a variable arc of rotation, depending on the incisions used near the base. Pedicle flaps based on the occipital vessels may be made lengthy with respect to their width because of the rich vascular supply that extends far anteriorly through the dermal and subdermal vascular plexuses.

All the scalp pedicles outlined in this section are carefully marked and measured for arc of rotation preoperatively. Because the scalp is thick and has strong attachments to the underlying galea, tension placed upon them does not gain appreciable length. Therefore, even defects in the scalp and skull that measure only a few square centimeters in area will require pedicle flaps that appear relatively large. In each case the scalp pedicle flap is elevated after incising its margins at the level of the galea, leaving the periosteum intact. This plane may be dissected easily, using blunt dissection, since no vascular structures traverse it from below. Preoperative palpation and use of a small Doppler vascular probe will outline the arterial system in each of the primary vascular territories. The scalp is shaved at that time and marked with indelible material such as Brilliant Green dye, which will remain after surgical preparation in the operating room.

SCALP ROTATION FLAPS

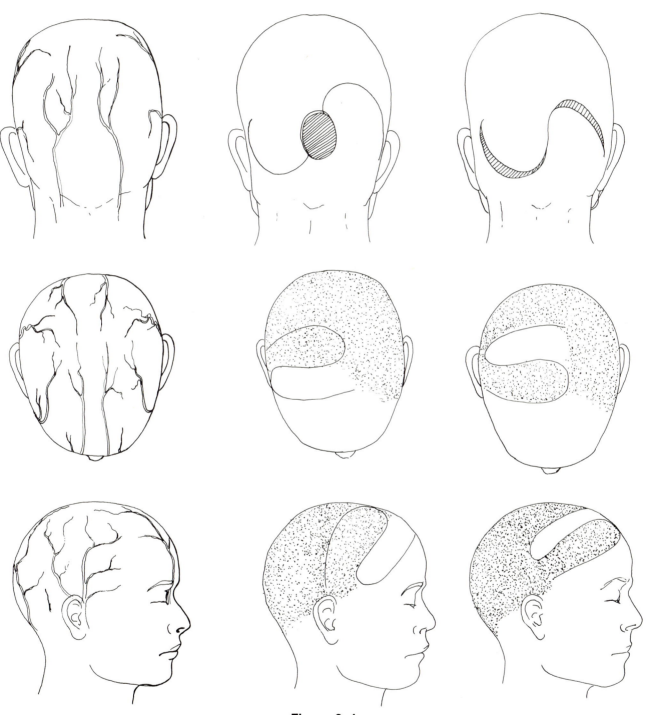

Figure 2-1

Figure 2–2. This patient sustained a scalp and superficial skull defect resulting from an electrical injury. The pericranium in the center of the defect was dessicated and would not support a split-thickness skin graft, although the peripheral margins of the wound consisted of healthy granulation tissue. Because of the deep central defect, pedicle flap coverage was chosen for reconstruction.

Figures 2–3, 2–4. The preoperative markings are indicated, including the arterial base at X: the right occipital artery. The cross-hatched area indicates the area of the pedicle that requires to be rotated laterally to cover the defect. Anteriorly, the resulting donor defect is estimated to facilitate the planning of a suitable split-thickness skin graft donor site.

Figure 2–5. The right occipital scalp flap is elevated. Neurosurgical skin clips are helpful to diminish bleeding from the edges of the scalp incisions. The wound has been debrided of granulation tissue

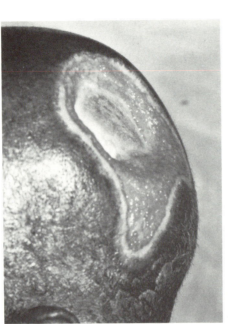

Figure 2–2

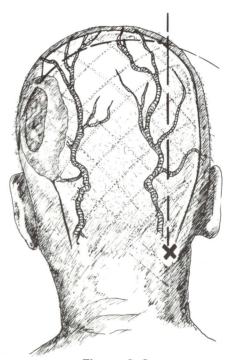

Figure 2–3

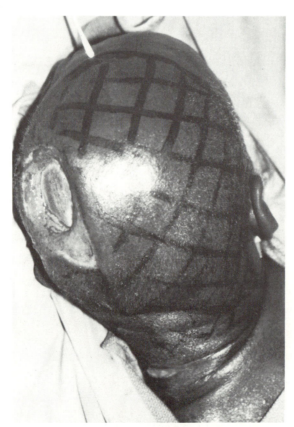

Figure 2–4

and desiccated pericranium over the outer table of the skull.

Figure 2–6. The arc of rotation of the scalp flap into the wound defect is demonstrated. In the event of a large "dog-ear" at the medial base of the flap, a small back-cut may be made with resection of a portion of the medial base of the flap, or of intact scalp over the adjacent skull. Any back-cut at the base of a scalp flap should not extend more than a distance equal to one-fourth of the width of the base. After a back-cut of that length, a residual "dog-ear" should be accepted rather than a further back-cut, which would compromise the blood supply to the flap. The "dog-ear" may be revised by excision several months later after primary healing of the transposed flap.

Figure 2–7. The transposed right occipital flap is sutured into position. A medium-thickness split skin graft (0.016 inches) is sutured into the resulting donor defect. A soft, pliable drain is placed beneath the transposed flap to avoid any hematoma collection under it that may compromise the venous drainage and lead to necrosis. A bulky, occlusive dressing is applied, and the patient is maintained in bed with his head elevated for two or three days after operation.

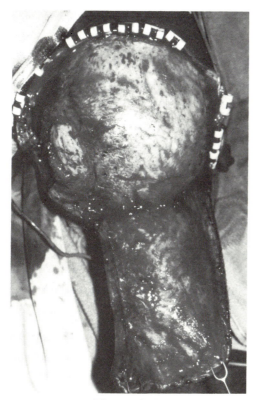

Figure 2-5

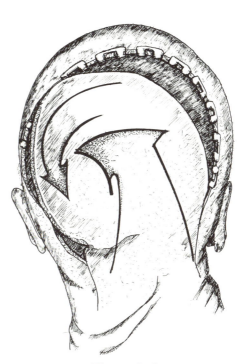

Figure 2-6

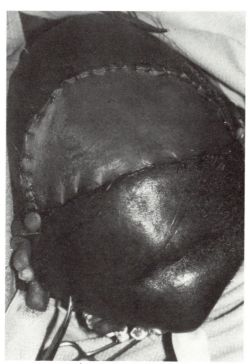

Figure 2-7

Figure 2–8. The left side of the patient's head is seen four weeks after surgery. The original wound site is completely covered with durable, well vascularized scalp.

Figures 2–9, 2–10. The posterior and right lateral portions of the scalp are seen several months later. In this elderly patient hair growth was sparse, both on the adjacent scalp and on the flap itself, so that camouflage of the skin graft was not possible.

Pitfalls and Solutions

1. Preoperative assessment of the vascular pedicle and of the arc of rotation possible with a particular scalp flap is mandatory. Estimation at the time of surgery without this preoperative assessment may result in a shortage of flap tissue, or in vascular compromise of a flap based in an area that has inadequate blood supply.

2. Back-cutting of the base of a scalp pedicle, away from the main arterial input, is permissible, but only for a distance usually one-fourth of the width of the total pedicle base. It is better to accept a fold or "dog-ear" at the time of surgery, which can be revised safely later, than to compromise the sole blood supply to the pedicle flap.

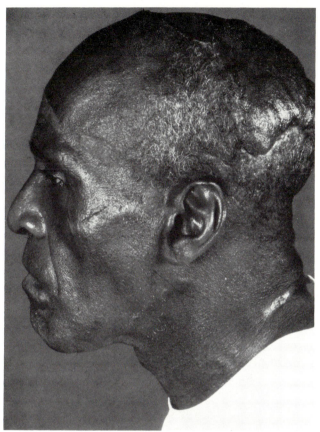

Figure 2-8

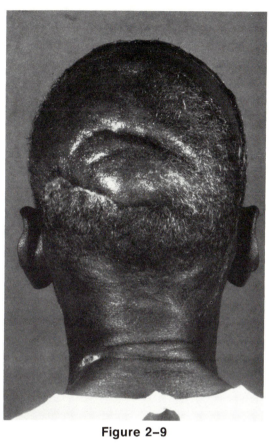

Figure 2-9

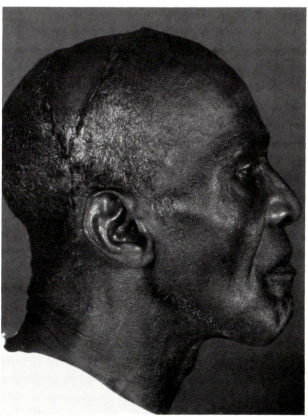

Figure 2-10

3

Visor Scalp Flap for Restoration of Anterior Hairline

The Problem

Loss of anterior hair-bearing scalp with obliteration of the hairline is common in facial burns. The resulting esthetic deformity is obvious and of great psychological import to the patient. The area of loss is often large in this region. Small, free "hair transplants" are inadequate because of poor vascularity of the recipient site, which leads to loss of many of the grafts. Further, the final appearance after multiple grafts of this type is often sparse and stubbly. For restoration of the hairline, especially when the area is large, a bipedicled "visor" scalp flap may be used.

Technique

Figures 3–1, 3–2. A young patient is shown with a large defect comprising the upper forehead, backward to the midvertex of the scalp.

Figure 3–3. The temporal scalp is richly supplied with branches of the superficial temporal artery. These branches course anteriorly and posteriorly, and approach the midline bilaterally.

Figure 3–4. Using palpation and a small Doppler vascular probe, the superficial temporal and posterior auricular arterial system can be marked preoperatively. The scalp should not be shaved closely, or landmarks may be partly obscured. Rather, the hair is clipped to a length of one-eighth of an inch prior to surgery.

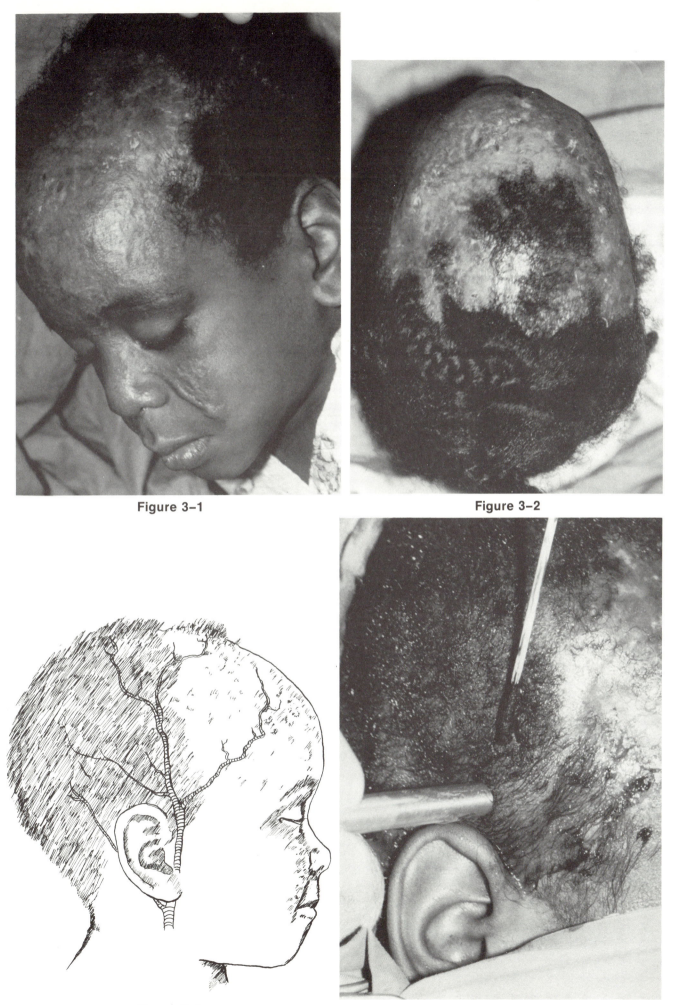

Figure 3-1

Figure 3-2

Figure 3-3

Figure 3-4

BURNS OF THE SCALP AND SKULL

Figure 3–5. The preoperative plan for this patient is outlined. The shaded area represents the portion of injured, hairless scalp to be excised, usually down to the level of the periosteum. The dotted lines indicate the anterior and posterior margins of the bipedicled "visor" flap, which is based on both superficial temporal arteries and their branches. The flap incisions are made down to the level of the intact galea. The dissection plane between the galea and the undersurface of the flap is quite bloodless, and is developed using blunt dissection. As the base of the flap on either side is approached, care is taken not to skeletonize the vascular structures entering the flap.

Figure 3–6. As the flap is elevated, it is intermittently moved forward to test the arc of rotation so that, when an adequate length is reached, there will be no tension upon the bases of the flap as it lies in its transposed position anteriorly. To achieve anterior mobility, the temporal incisions may be carefully extended posteriorly, avoiding injury to any posterior arterial branches supplying the flap.

Figure 3–7. The bipedicled flap is advanced anteriorly to cover the defect. It is sutured into place by peripheral, interrupted 5-0 monofilament sutures. Hemostasis is secured by electrocoagulation of bleeding points along the periphery of the flap, to avoid hematoma formation that would lead to internal pressure, possibly enough to interfere with its blood supply. A medium-thickness, split-thickness skin graft (or grafts) (0.014- to 0.018-inch) is removed from a suitable donor area and sutured into the defect left by the transposition of the flap, using 5-0 monofilament or synthetic, absorbable suture material. A soft, bulky dressing is placed over the entire scalp for protection. The margins and surface of the bipedicled flap may be examined by gently elevating the dressing periodically during the first two days after surgery, to ensure that no interference with the flap's blood supply has occurred.

Figures 3–8, 3–9, 3–10. The early initial healing of the flap and skin graft covering the donor defect is shown.

Pitfalls and Solutions

1. Preoperative assessment of the superficial temporal arterial vascular territory is mandatory to avoid transposing a flap that may be ischemic from the start.

2. The "visor" flap can be made as narrow as from 5 to 8 cm or as wide as 10 to 15 cm in most patients. Preoperative marking and assessment of the size requirements will avoid compromise of the result by a flap of incorrect dimensions.

3. Pressure at the bases of the flap by an ill-fitting dressing must be avoided. Frequent postoperative inspection of the flap is required.

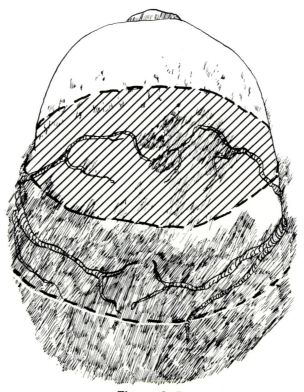

Figure 3–5

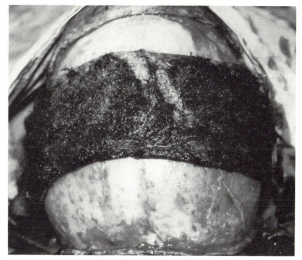
Figure 3-6

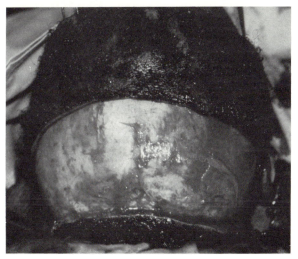
Figure 3-7

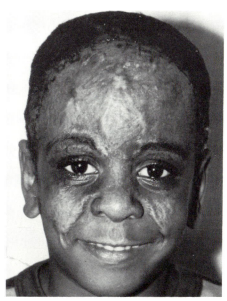
Figure 3-8

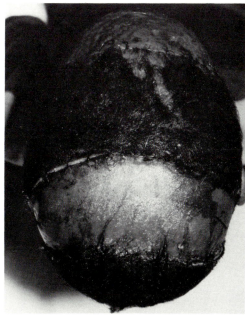
Figure 3-9

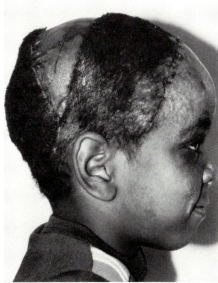
Figure 3-10

4

Loss of the Scalp and Destruction of The Underlying Pericranium

The Problem

When injury that has caused loss of the scalp and pericranium occurs, the underlying skull will sequester to varying degrees. Split-thickness skin grafts will appear to heal over beds of granulation tissue that had responded to the local injury. Granulation tissue that develops in this manner has a considerable resorptive capacity with respect to the underlying bone. It is often noted that even intact, initially viable skull underlying granulation tissue will undergo loss of integrity, become softened and demineralized, and eventually sequester. This process can also occur after skin grafts applied to the granulation tissue have healed. It is not possible to predict which patient will heal in this manner, without bony sequestration, and which patient will require a later, secondary reconstructive procedure.

Technique

Figures 4–1, 4–2. A patient aged two years has lost the scalp and underlying pericranium from a thermal injury. Portions of the outer table of the skull are locally damaged, but the inner table is intact.

Figure 4–3. The diploë are exposed, with preservation of the intact inner table of the skull. By use of a neurosurgical burr, holes are placed over the entire surface of the injured skull, entering the diploë, but not damaging the inner table. From these areas of diploë granulation tissue will develop, and over a period of several days will coalesce to cover the remaining areas of exposed skull. The granulation tissue in this instance acts as a neovascular bed or recipient site for split-thickness skin grafts.

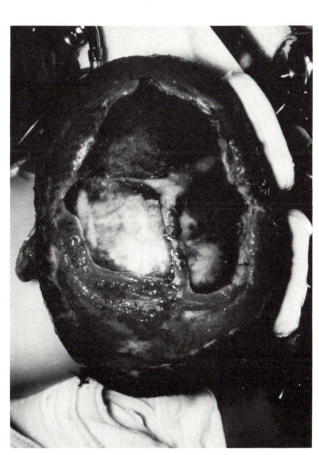

Figure 4-1

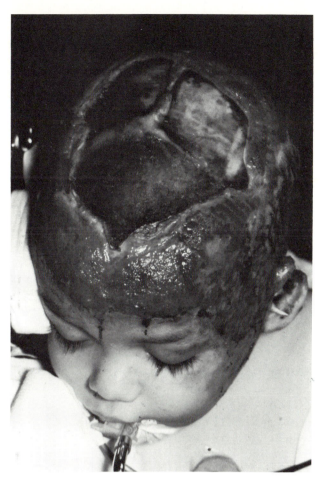

Figure 4-2

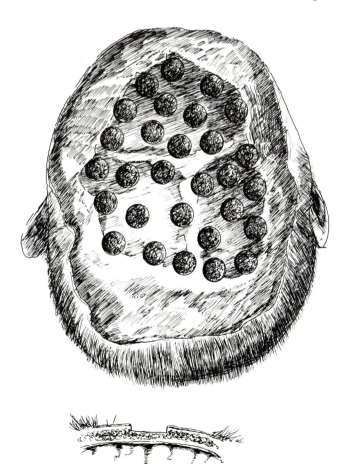

Figure 4-3

Figures 4–4, 4–5. Large, medium-thickness (0.014- to 0.018-inch) skin grafts are applied to the recipient bed of granulation tissue, and dressed with occlusive bandages. Although early healing is the rule, it is not possible to predict whether or not this initial procedure will be definitive, or if a later revision will be required if sequestration of the underlying skull occurs.

Careful observation of the patient continues for as long as the grafts remain viable and provide durable, healed coverage of the skull. Roentgenograms of the skull are obtained if there is any suspicion of the development of an underlying pathologic condition.

Figures 4–6, 4–7. The same patient is seen eight years after surgery and application of split-thickness skin grafts to the resulting granulation tissue recipient site. No further operative procedures were required, and with an esthetically suitable hair piece this patient achieved a reasonable appearance.

Pitfalls and Solutions

1. Burr holes must be made carefully so that injury to the inner table of the skull, and especially to the underlying dura, is avoided. With defects over the vertex of the skull, in particular, penetration through the dura may produce massive fetal hemorrhage from the underlying sagittal sinus.

2. A patient treated with skin grafts over a neovascular bed of granulation tissue in the manner described must be followed and observed frequently for a very prolonged period. He (or his family) must be apprised of the possible necessity of a later, secondary reconstructive procedure in the event of sequestration of the underlying skull.

LOSS OF THE SCALP AND DESTRUCTION OF THE UNDERLYING PERICRANIUM

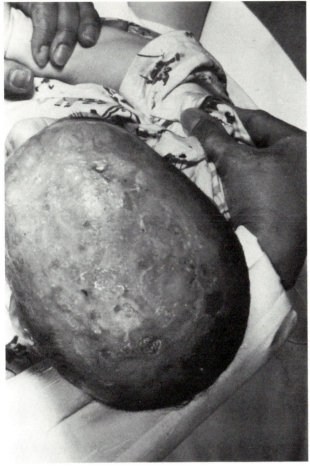

Figure 4-4

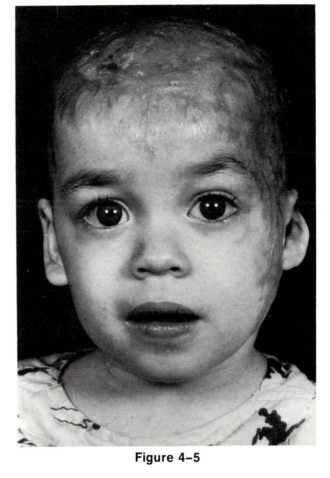

Figure 4-5

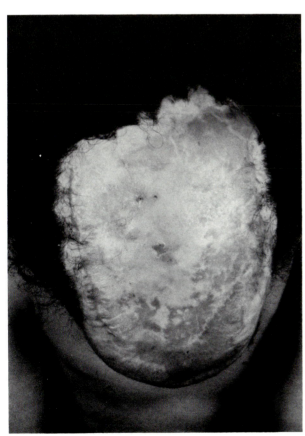

Figure 4-6

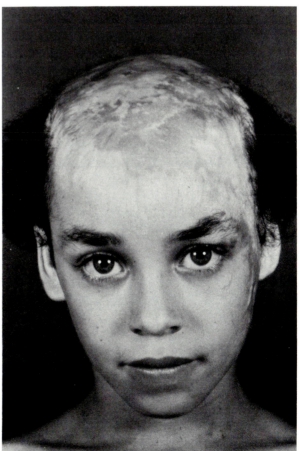

Figure 4-7

5

Loss of the Scalp and Underlying Skull: Decortication

The Problem

Loss of the scalp and underlying full-thickness skull can occur in several ways. Direct injury, often from electrical burns, can initially destroy all of the tissues external to the brain. Even after coverage of the skull when only the pericranium is initially destroyed, sequestration of the skull can ensue. In either event it may become necessary to decorticate the damaged skull and provide durable, vascularized coverage, to achieve prolonged wound healing and protection of the brain.

Technique

Figure 5–1. This patient sustained exposed, nonviable skull at the vertex following an electrical injury. An initial skin graft was applied after small drill holes had been made through the outer table into the diploë, and a granulation tissue bed was produced. Early healing was adequate, but over a period of two years areas of the skin graft became chronically ulcerated. Roentgenograms revealed sequestration and demineralization of the underlying full thickness of the skull.

Figure 5–2. A method of decortication of skull in the wound area is shown. A high-speed circular saw is used to divide the area of damaged skull into small squares or rectangles. Care must be taken to apply gentle pressure and to test the depth of the saw cut frequently, to avoid injury or penetration of the dura. This is particularly important over the vertex of the skull, because of the proximity of the underlying sagittal venous sinus. Penetration into the sagittal sinus can result in massive, fatal hemorrhage.

The cross-sectional view of the skull after the several saw cuts have been made reveals a matrix of small, rectangular islands of skull. A blunt, curved periosteal elevator is used to gently explore the undersurface of each island, carefully elevating it from the underlying dura. Using cautious side-to-side dissection, each island is gradually lifted and removed.

The process of elevation and removal is repeated for each of the several skull islands. Irregular areas at the periphery of the resulting skull defect are smoothed and further excised, using a bone rongeur. The vascularity of the diploë at the edge of the skull defect is assessed, and resection of bone continues until adequate vascularity is noted.

Figure 5–3. After decortication in the manner described, the dura is exposed in the central portion of the wound, with the sagittal sinus lying beneath. It was necessary in this case to rongeur additional bone, extending the resection beneath the viable scalp in some areas. Because of the size and location of this particular defect, coverage with a local vascular pedicle flap of scalp was chosen. A large, long pedicle of occipital scalp was incised and elevated. The flap is raised at the level of the galea, leaving the periosteum beneath intact.

The pedicle flap is rotated into the defect over the vertex. Multiple sutures of 4-0 monofilament material are used to maintain the position of the flap. A medium-thickness (0.014-inch) skin graft is taken and sutured into the flap donor site. A drain was employed beneath the flap to avoid hematoma, and an occlusive dressing was applied, care being taken not to constrict the base of the pedicle flap. Following surgery the patient is maintained in bed for three or four days, with the head of the bed elevated to assist dependent drainage of the flap. The drain can be removed by the second postoperative day. Hair growth from the adjacent scalp and from the transposed flap is usually adequate to camouflage a donor defect of this size.

Pitfalls and Solutions

1. Injury to the dura and any underlying vascular sinus must be avoided. Neurosurgical consultation should be requested to assist in decortication if the operator is inexperienced in this technique, or if there is any doubt concerning a pathologic condition (such as brain abscess) beneath the skull.

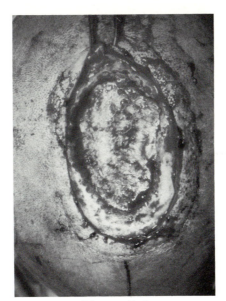

Figure 5–1

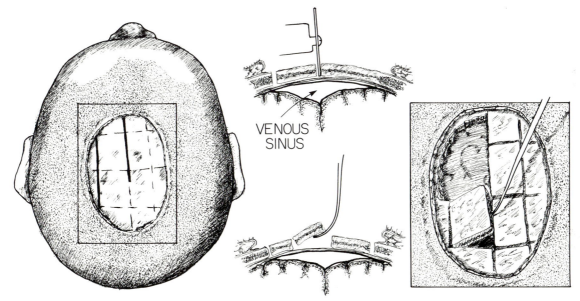

Figure 5–2

VENOUS SINUS

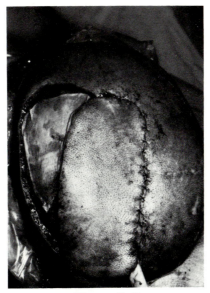

Figure 5–3

Reconstruction of the Thermally Injured Ear

Reconstruction of the thermally injured ear has a low priority because it is rarely an isolated injury, but often part of a far more extensive burn involving the visible areas of the face. McIndoe estimated an average of 25 operations for patients with burned faces in his series. It should be obvious to both the patient and the surgeon that a part that can be camouflaged by allowing the hair to grow long or using a hair piece should be reconstructed last. In fact, many individuals refuse offers of surgical correction.

The most common deformities are:
a. Total loss due to initial injury or a subsequent bacterial infection.
b. Partial or complete helical loss.
c. A contracted and deformed lobule.

The number of patients with total loss of the ear amenable to reconstruction is indeed small. Unlike those with microtia, in whom the normal anatomy is lacking but the surrounding and intrinsic tissues are uninjured, burned patients often have dense scar that is unyielding to the surgeon's attempts at resculpturing. For the occasional individual who desires total reconstruction, the reader is referred to the excellent and very complete writings of Tanzer, Converse, and Brent. For the patient who refuses surgery, options are the use of a toupee; increased hair length; or prosthetic ears. These last have a very checkered reputation because prostheses do not tolerate the abuse that an active, playing child will challenge them with, and become conspicuous since they do not respond with seasonal changes in color as do normal skin areas.

6

Reconstruction of the Superior Helix by Retroauricular Skin Advancement

The Problem

Many different flaps are described for superior helix reconstruction, and yield satisfactory results. This technique is a simple one when cartilages are intact and the soft tissue defect is localized.

Technique

Figure 6–1. Superior helix skin and soft tissue are thin and atrophic, but postauricular skin is intact and unscarred. Significantly, the helical cartilage is present in its entirety, and soft tissue coverage of the rest of the ear is very satisfactory.

Figure 6–2. A retroauricular incision is outlined over the mastoid process, extending from the superior part of the helix to the level of the external meatus.

Figure 6–3A, B. Following infiltration of local anesthetic with epinephrine, a relatively bloodless plane is achieved. Dissection on perichondrium must be carried anteriorly to fully mobilize the skin for advancement.

Figure 6–4. The skin is advanced and redraped, creating a new helical border, and held in its new position with several mattress sutures placed through anterior skin, cartilage, and posterior skin. The retroauricular skin defect can be closed with a skin graft, or by mobilization and advancement of the posterior scalp. The ear dressing must be applied meticulously to avoid any pressure point, since the blood supply of the skin is tenuous, and pressure necrosis may result.

Figure 6–5. There is now fullness of the superior helix.

Pitfalls and Solutions

Blood supply to the healed burn is often tenuous, and so the plane of dissection must be on cartilage when the soft tissue and skin are elevated.

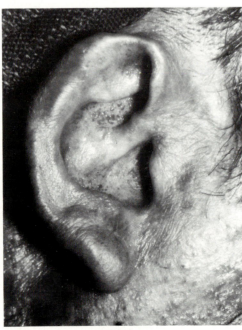

Figure 6–1

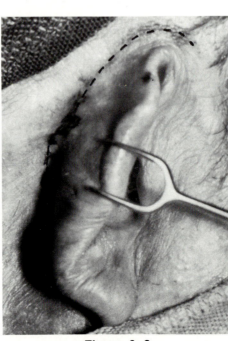

Figure 6–2

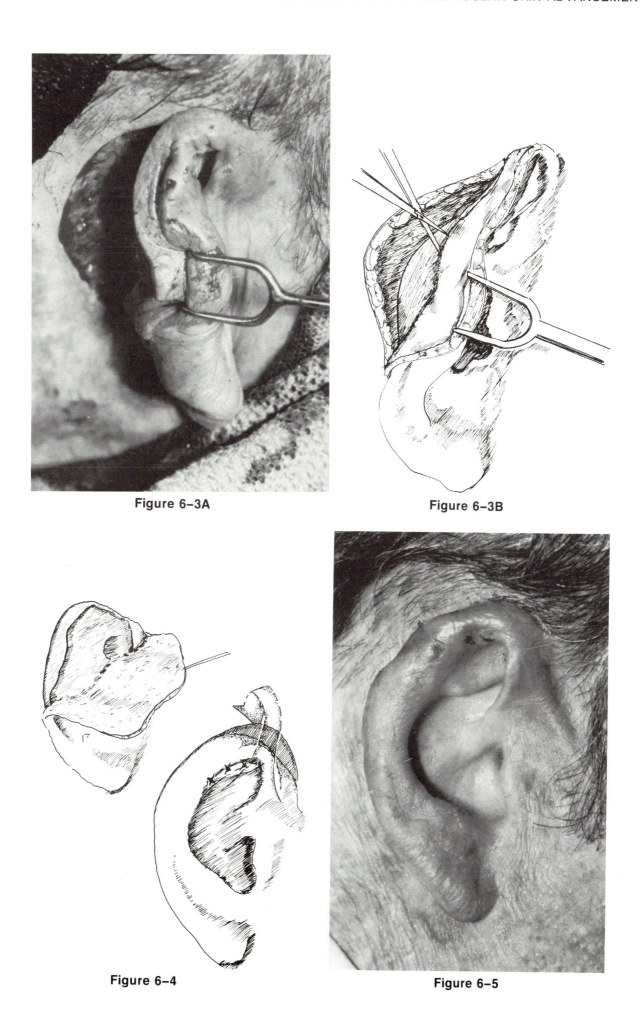

Figure 6-3A

Figure 6-3B

Figure 6-4

Figure 6-5

7

Cartilage Defect of the Superior Helix

The Problem

Moderate loss of cartilage can be managed by local flaps with implantation of cartilage, or by mobilization of existing ear. Advancement of the entire helix, as described by Antia, provides a solution that utilizes local tissue. Although the total ear size is somewhat reduced with this technique, the result can be pleasing and proportional.

Technique

Figure 7–1. An ear is illustrated in which there has been moderate loss of cartilage as well as of soft tissue from the superior helix.

Figure 7–2. Prospective skin incisions are marked. Note that the inferior portion of the incision passes over the tail of the helix, and continues to the very apex of the helix.

Figure 7–3A, B. Superiorly, the skin and cartilage are incised. The resulting pedicle is elevated as a flap and shifted inferiorly. An inferior incision is made through anterior skin and cartilage. The tail of the helix is cut and the antihelical skin is mobilized, allowing the pedicle to move superiorly. If mobilization is not complete, forcing this segment superiorly will result in a cup-shaped ear. The margins of the advanced flap are incised to expose cartilage edges, which are sutured to each other. The cartilage is joined with interrupted 5-0 synthetic, absorbable sutures, and the skin approximated with interrupted 5-0 monofilament suture.

Figure 7–4. Two weeks postoperatively the incisions are healing, but a small ulcer secondary to ischemia has developed.

Figure 7–5. Slight notching at the cartilage juncture because of wound contraction has precluded an optimal result.

Pitfalls and Solutions

1. All tissues in the healed, burned ear are fragile, and often have marginal blood supply. Reconstruction with advancement flaps such as these are tenuous, and some tissue loss may occur.

2. Intraoperatively, buckling of the antihelix may result because of the length of the advancement flaps in the patient with a large defect. This will not smooth out with time, but instead will result in a cup-ear deformity. If buckling of the antihelix occurs at surgery, a wedge-shaped piece of conchal cartilage should be excised, giving a smooth appearance and a natural-looking ear.

CARTILAGE DEFECT OF THE SUPERIOR HELIX

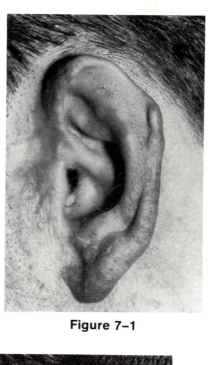

Figure 7-1

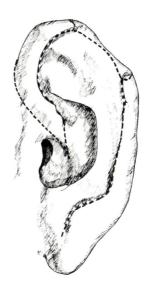

Figure 7-2

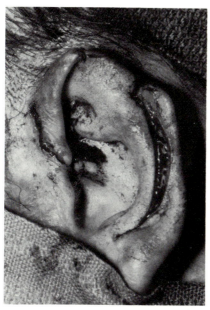

Figure 7-3A

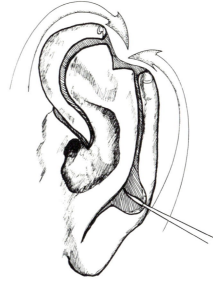

Figure 7-3B

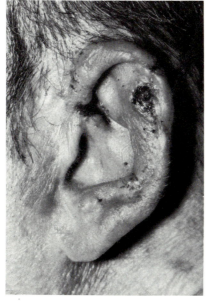

Figure 7-4

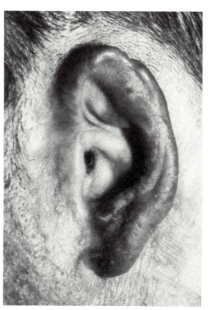

Figure 7-5

29

8

The Contracted Ear Lobule

The Problem

Figure 8–1. Loss of lobule identity is common when the burn injury involves the adjoining cheek, resulting in a bridging scar. Local flaps such as Z-plasty or V-Y advancement under local anesthesia offer a simple solution with minimal tissue manipulation.

Technique

Figure 8–2. A Z-plasty is outlined to release the linear contraction and produce a rounded lobule.

Figure 8–3. The flaps are transposed and most of the tension is removed from the lobule, but lobule configuration is still not correct.

Figure 8–4. A single, triangular advancement flap is cut that outlines the inferior pole of the lobule. The flap is moved posteriorly and sutured in place. The cut ends of the lobule are sutured to each other, and lobule definition is achieved.

Figure 8–5. Satisfactory lobule definition is seen one year postoperatively.

Pitfalls and Solutions

When planning the flap reconstruction, the surgeon must be sure that the proposed flap will move superiorly and backward rather than anteriorly, or the lobule may be cupped forward in a very unnatural position.

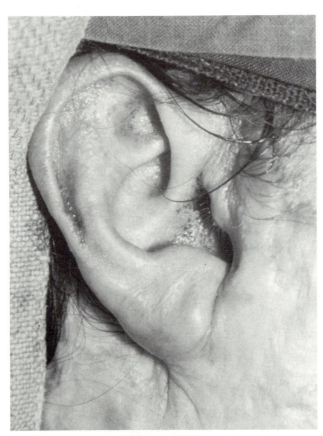

Figure 8–1

THE CONTRACTED EAR LOBULE

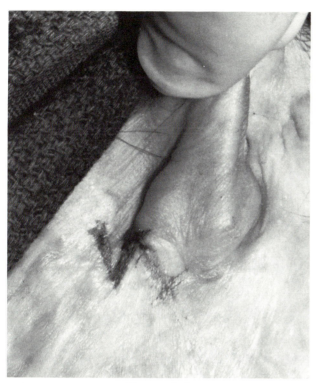

Figure 8-2

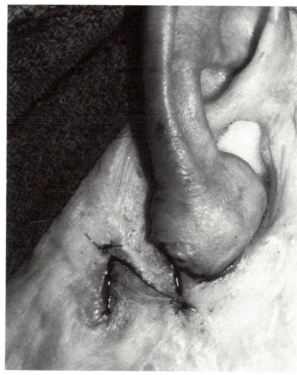

Figure 8-3

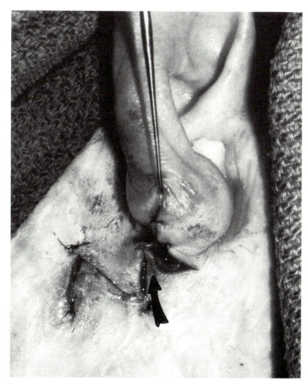

Figure 8-4

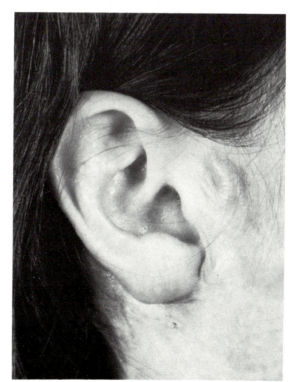

Figure 8-5

31

Burns of the Face

Even the most gifted surgeon may be thwarted in reconstructing deep second- and third-degree burns of the face because of tissue destruction. For the surgeon lacking formal art training or an understanding of the basic tenets of anatomical proportion, the task is impossible. Since it is rare for only one feature to be involved and the rest of the face spared, a knowledge of anatomical relationships is very important.

The choice of procedures for restoring the integrity of esthetic facial units includes multiple partial excisions, grafts, or pedicles. Partial excision is useful in the adult with redundant skin, but less so in the child in whom distortion of features may result. Grafts may be full- or split-thickness, from the supraclavicular area, neck, or scalp. Split-thickness skin grafts from below the clavicle have the disadvantage of a poor color match, especially in the case of skin from the abdomen, which often becomes yellow with time. Tattooing of this skin has not been particularly successful. Pedicle coverage is useful for building structures that have been destroyed, such as the nose, but not for replacing skin loss, because of the masklike face that results. Intimate attachment of muscle to skin is lost if a flap is used, and although the appearance may be reasonable in repose, the patient cannot animate it and expression is impossible.

9

Anatomical Imperatives and Esthetic Facial Units: The Art of Seeing

Figure 9–1. Although the face is seen as a whole, in an adult it is artistically divided into thirds:

Hairline to root of nose — one-third.
Root of nose to base of columella — one-third.
Base of columella to tip of chin — one-third.

The width of each eye is usually equal to the distance between the inner canthi, which is also equal to the distance between the alar rims. The mouth commissures are located at the upper third of the distance between the nose and the chin, and its width is about equal to the inner limbus distance. The ear resides on a plane between the root of the nose and the columellar base. An imaginary horizontal line (Frankfort) should pass through the infraorbital rim and superior external auditory canal. Lastly, the length of the auricle is about two times its width. It is important to remember these relationships because injuries are often bilateral, and one cannot copy a normal side when there is none.

The face is rarely symmetrical, but is seen as such by the viewer unless there is obvious deformity. Thus, any patchwork within a facial unit arrests the eye, destroys the image of the whole, and is discordant. Occasionally it is best to sacrifice normal tissue to restore the image of the whole.

Figure 9–2. Multiple hypertrophic burn scars above the lip are present, but nearly half of the tissue between the nasolabial folds is unburned. Limited excision and closures would produce distortion, and possibly worse scarring; closure by excision and multiple small grafts would create a "spotted Dalmatian" effect.

Figure 9–3. Excision of all tissue between the nasolabial folds is planned, with suture lines placed in the folds, commissures of the mouth, and border of the upper lip. Scalp skin is used to resurface the defect.

Figure 9–4. The result is pleasingly smooth and unobtrusive. Some believe that a keloid former such as this child is no candidate for surgery, but, following the concept of unit replacement, many suture lines can be either hidden or placed in natural creases. Thus, the thickened scars that may develop in spite of fine technique and steroid injections are at least in normal creases.

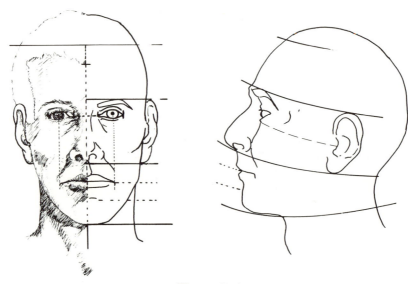

Figure 9–1

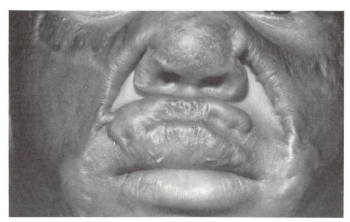

Figure 9-2

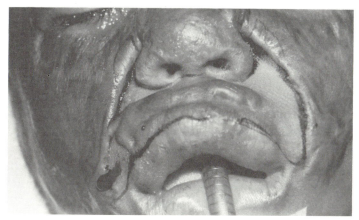

Figure 9-3

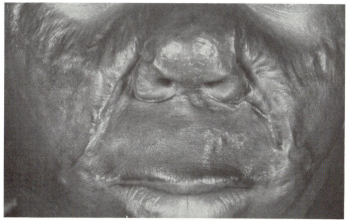

Figure 9-4

BURNS OF THE FACE

The esthetic facial units are:
Figure 9–5. Forehead.
Figure 9–6. Chin, lower lip.
Figure 9–7. Upper lip.
Figure 9–8. Eyelids, periorbita.
Figure 9–9. Cheeks, nose.

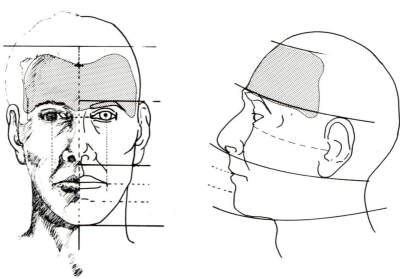

Figure 9–5

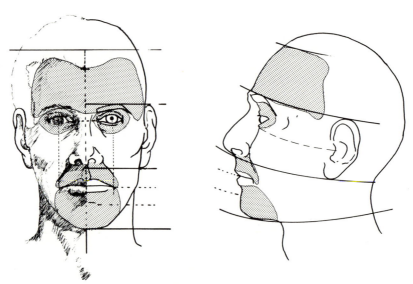

Figure 9–6

ANATOMICAL IMPERATIVES AND ESTHETIC FACIAL UNITS: THE ART OF SEEING

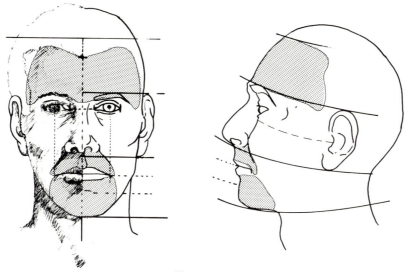

Figure 9-7

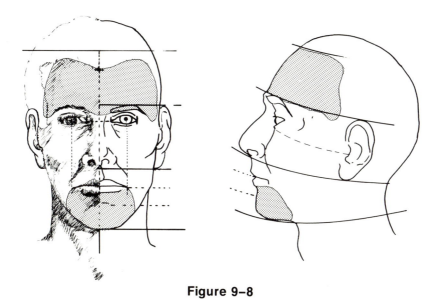

Figure 9-8

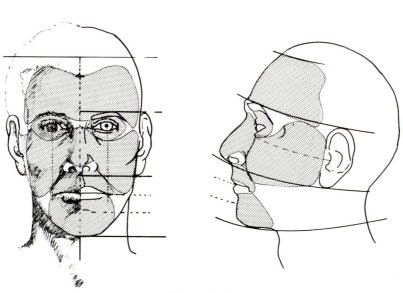

Figure 9-9

Figure 9–10. Management of the upper unit of the face (forehead) usually gives an excellent result with one split-thickness sheet graft, the suture lines following hair, eyebrows, and lateral canthi to the ears. Later, the hair can be combed forward to hide the incision. This particular patient had a third-degree burn of the entire face, and every esthetic unit was grafted as indicated by the Brilliant Green markings.

In the middle third of the face the viewer's attention is usually arrested by the eyes, and then moves to the cheeks and ears. The ears have the lowest priority, and can be concealed by a Prince Valiant haircut or even a wig.

Figure 9–11. The cheeks may not have a perfect color match, and yet will look excellent if graft is carried to the lower eyelid skin superiorly, medially to the nasolabial folds, laterally to the preauricular creases, and inferiorly to the mandible. This butterfly pattern tends to be less obtrusive than postage stamp grafting patches of healed second-degree burn.

Priorities of Reconstruction

The priorities of reconstruction depend on whether the problems are functional, esthetic, or both.

Figure 9–12. Severe lower lid ectropion with chronic conjunctivitis or drooling from a lower lip contracted to the sternum would warrant the earliest correction, whereas the rebuilding of a helical rim might be done last.

The plan for sequential reconstruction of facial units is more than academic if good donor skin is limited. The most visible units should be covered with the best color-matched skin. Thus, one might proceed in the following order:

a. Eyelids.
b. Lips.
c. Cheeks.
d. Chin.
e. Nose.
f. Eyebrows.
g. Forehead.
h. Scalp.

Donor Site Selection

The donor site is very important in achieving an overall pleasing effect, as juxtaposing skin from different areas may create a zebra-like effect. Although some surgeons have taken into account thickness of skin in choosing a donor site, it is the color that is most important when selecting coverage for esthetic units of the face. The best color match is achieved with skin above the clavicle, and this can be taken by distending the supraclavicular area with saline to create a large, flat surface for removing grafts with a small drum dermatome. The scalp also can be shaved and injected with saline. The color match is superb, as is the skin quality. The initial reluctance to shave the head is quickly lost when one sees that the results are excellent and that no donor sites are visible. Because large sheets of skin can be harvested from the scalp, it is excellent for resurfacing the eyelid, being thin and of good color. If the head is burned and the surgeon must go below the clavicles, it is wise to use the same donor site to cover a whole area. For instance, the abdomen and buttocks can be donors for the chin, nose, and cheeks. Even though the skin may become yellow, it is easier to match the color with cosmetics than if multiple adjoining areas of different color are used.

ANATOMICAL IMPERATIVES AND ESTHETIC FACIAL UNITS: THE ART OF SEEING

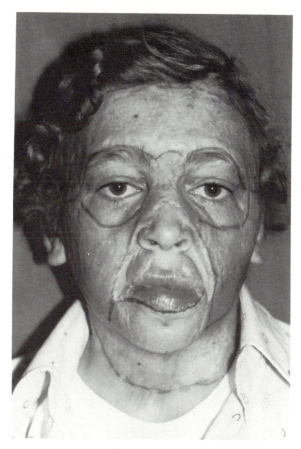

Figure 9-10

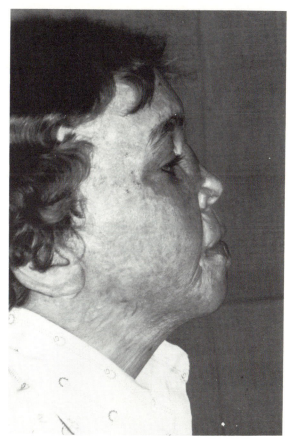

Figure 9-11

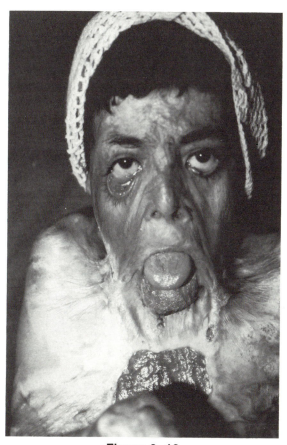

Figure 9-12

10

The Eyebrow: Total and Partial Loss

The Problem

Loss of portions of the eyebrows may occur with facial burn injury. Total loss of the eyebrows is uncommon, but when this happens it results in an obvious esthetic defect that is difficult to camouflage with only surface cosmetics. The use of such cosmetics may be particularly disturbing for male patients.

Technique

When the temporal scalp and underlying superficial temporal artery are present, total eyebrow replacement is possible using an island pedicle flap of scalp.

Figure 10–1. The general anatomy of an island scalp flap in the temporal region is illustrated. Using palpation and a small Doppler blood flow probe, the course of the superficial temporal artery and its branches may be marked on the scalp preoperatively. The temporal scalp is shaved, and a template of the contralateral normal eyebrow (if present) can be made by tracing the normal contours on sterile, transparent plastic material. This template is positioned over the site for the new eyebrow, and its outline marked. General anesthesia is ordinarily used for the surgical procedure, but local anesthesia is possible in selected patients. If local anesthetics are used, epinephrine should not be added, or vasospasm of the arterial pedicle may result.

An incision over the main proximal course of the superficial temporal artery is made, and carried superiorly. The arc of rotation from the proximal artery, anterior to the ear, to the recipient site is measured. The template is then used to outline the donor scalp contour. After exposing the superficial temporal artery through the initial incision, superior to the point of the scalp island, the dissection continues at a level just above the temporal fascia. No attempt is made to skeletonize completely the vascular pedicle to the scalp flap; this might result in injury to the vascular supply. An enveloping layer of soft tissue should be left around the vascular pedicle to the point of entry into the scalp flap. The scalp island is elevated from the temporal fascia, and small, peripheral bleeding points are ligated with fine, absorbable suture material.

Figure 10–2. A subcutaneous tunnel is created, extending from the proximal portion of the temporal incision anteriorly to the site of the new eyebrow. Using the template once again, a full-thickness excision of the scar in this region is carried out in the following manner.

The periphery of the contour of the new eyebrow is incised deeply. The scar is dissected from the borders of the new wound in such a way as to leave two parallel, V-shaped grooves along the course of the base of the excision site *(a)*. In cross-section, the base of the excision site then has the appearance of a "W." This will create a maximal surface area for the island pedicle to make contact with, and enhance effective cross-circulation between the pedicle flap and the recipient site. After completing this excision, the subcutaneous tunnel is widened and connected with the dissection at the proximal vascular base of the pedicle flap. The island scalp pedicle is passed carefully through the tunnel, avoiding kinking or torsion of the pedicle. Once in place, the island portion is turned over, and a shallow incision 1 to 1.5 mm deep is made in the center of the subcutaneous surface of the flap, avoiding major vessels, *A*. This will allow the flap to fit over the W-shaped excision wound, *A–(a)*. Aside from maximizing surface contact, this will permit the peripheral margins to be sutured so that the flap will lie in a somewhat concave position. When new hair growth occurs, over several weeks, the hairs will intertwine, much as is the case with a normal eyebrow. Unless this fitting of the flap is done in the manner described, the new hairs are likely to have a vertical, "crew-cut" appearance that is unlike a normal eyebrow.

Figure 10–3. After suturing the flap into place with 6-0 monofilament material, the scalp donor incision is closed with 5-0 sutures.

THE EYEBROW: TOTAL AND PARTIAL LOSS

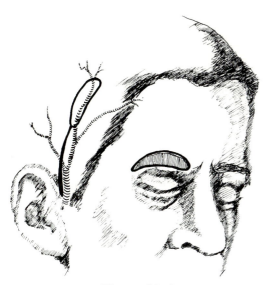

Figure 10-1

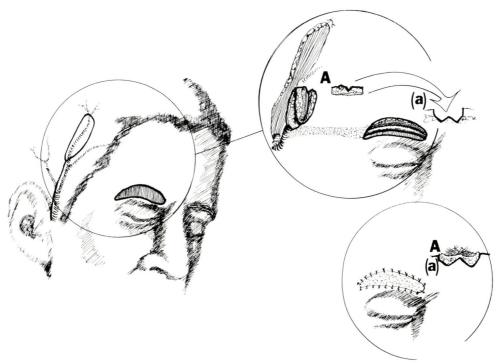

Figure 10-2

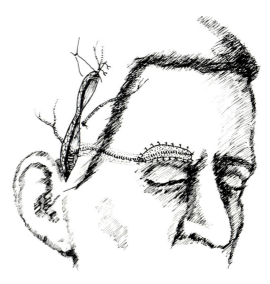

Figure 10-3

41

BURNS OF THE FACE

Figures 10–4, 10–5. A patient is shown in whom an island scalp pedicle was used to replace a missing left eyebrow by the method described. It is important to indicate to the patient that spontaneous epilation may occur after some initial regrowth of hair is noted, and may last several weeks. With return of hair growth, no further epilation occurs. The patient must trim the eyebrow hair occasionally, since it grows at the rate of scalp hair, which is faster than normal eyebrow hair growth. If both eyebrows are missing, templates are made taking into account the individual patient's orbital and facial anatomy.

Partial losses of the eyebrow(s) can be managed by using free, full-thickness, hair-bearing scalp grafts.

Figure 10–6. This patient sustained loss of the lateral third of the left eyebrow, and other facial burns.

Figure 10–7. The excision site marked over the area of the lateral eyebrow is indicated. (A reconstructive procedure for the malar eminence was performed at this same operative session.)

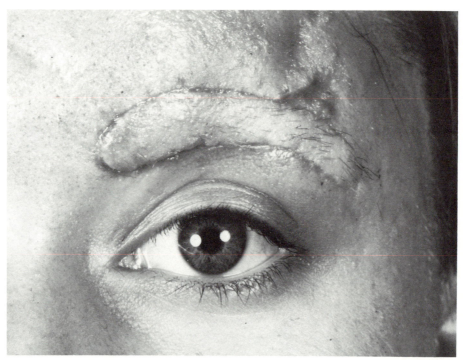

Figure 10–4

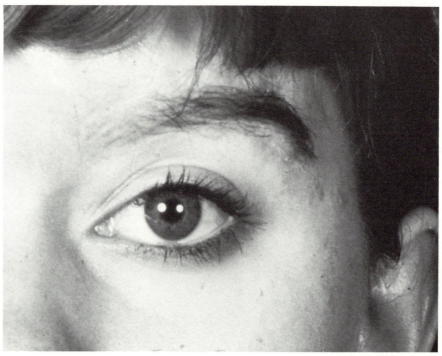

Figure 10–5

THE EYEBROW: TOTAL AND PARTIAL LOSS

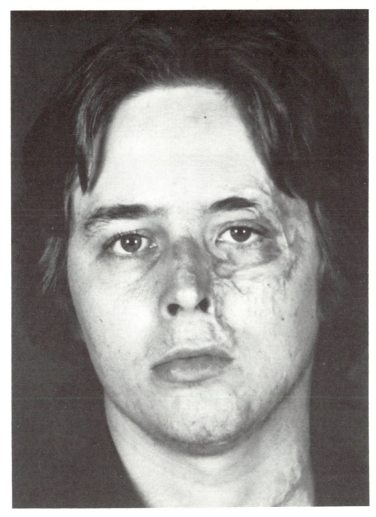

Figure 10-6

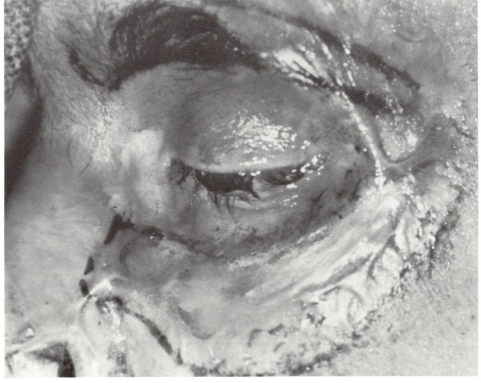

Figure 10-7

Figure 10–8. The temporal scalp is chosen for the donor site for grafts because the hairs lie flat, and drape inferiorly. When the graft is taken and rotated 90 degrees in the new brow position, the hairs will also lie flat, but laterally, as is the case with normal brow hairs. The free graft is excised just above the level of the temporal fascia. The excision site is made with a cross-sectional W-shape, and the free graft is incised on its deep surface in the same way as described for the island scalp flap technique. Occipital scalp may be used in the same manner, since the hairs there lie in the proper position, much like those in a normal eyebrow.

Figure 10–9. The donor defect extends to the temporal fascia. This incision is closed with 5-0 monofilament sutures.

Figure 10–10. The free scalp graft is sutured into position at the lateral brow area with fine, interrupted 6-0 monofilament sutures, so that a minimum of hair follicles are affected by the suture.

Figure 10–11. Two years following surgery, the patient has reasonable contour and fullness of the left eyebrow. Any disparity between the two eyebrows may be corrected by selectively plucking hair from either brow, or by means of a cosmetic eyebrow pencil.

Pitfalls and Solutions

1. Epinephrine must not be used in the region of island scalp pedicles because of the possibility of causing ischemia secondary to vasospasm.

2. Injury to the vascular pedicle to the island scalp flap must be prevented during dissection. No skeletonization of the vessels is required; this would be dangerous. A surrounding cuff of soft tissue is left intact about the vascular pedicle.

3. Passage of the island pedicle flap through the subcutaneous tunnel must be done without kinking it or causing tension on the vessels, either of which could lead to ischemia and necrosis of the scalp flap tissue.

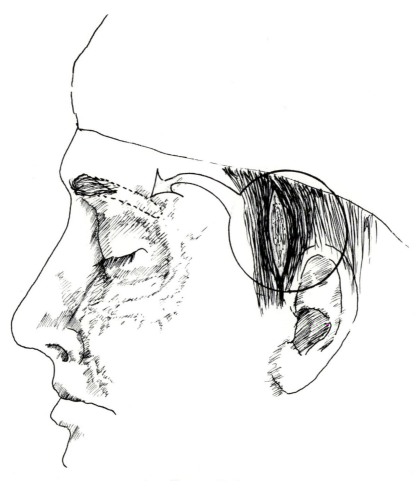

Figure 10–8

THE EYEBROW: TOTAL AND PARTIAL LOSS

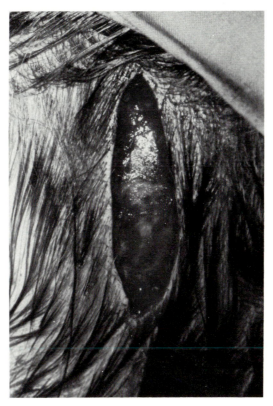

Figure 10-9

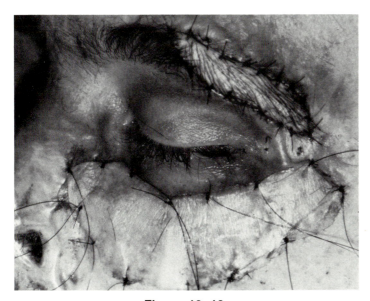

Figure 10-10

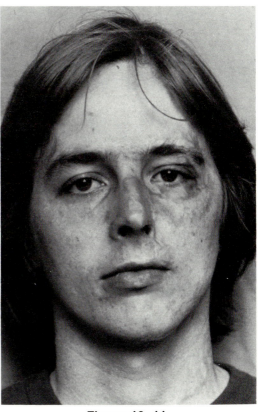

Figure 10-11

11

Upper Eyelid Ectropion

The Problem

Ectropion of the upper lid is less common than that of the lower lid, and may be corrected electively. If it is so severe that there is lack of corneal protection, surgical intervention is demanded.

Figure 11–1. Preoperative preparation must include a review of the anatomy of the levator mechanism, or a severe postoperative iatrogenic defect may result. The drawing illustrates the ease with which the insertion of the levator could be cut if an inappropriate incision were made. Specifically, the levator inserts not only into the tarsus but also into the eyelid skin. The incision must be sited above the normal sulcus of the eyelid.

Technique

Figure 11–2. In this patient, who is attempting to shut his eyes, it is obvious that there is a shortening of the upper lid. The prospective incision is outlined with methylene blue, extending from the medial to the lateral canthus and obliquely upward into a "crow's-foot." The arch of the incision is high enough to avoid damage to the levator muscle.

Figure 11–3. The incision extends through the subcutaneous tissue and fibers of the orbicularis to achieve a complete release. The medial extent of the incision divides the vertical scar band between the nose and the canthi. A medium-thickness skin graft (0.018-inch) is used for the upper lid reconstruction.

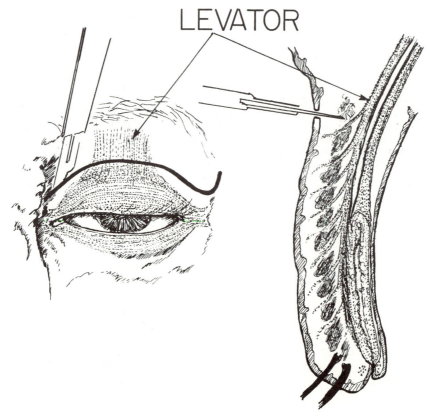

Figure 11–1

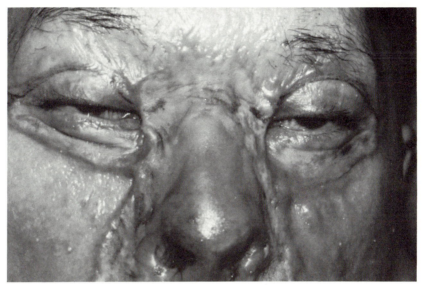

Figure 11-2

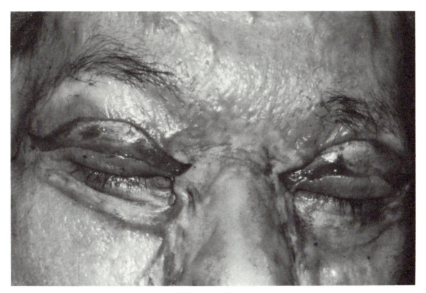

Figure 11-3

BURNS OF THE FACE

Figures 11–4, 11–5. With the patient looking upward or closing his eyes, it is obvious that the release of both lids has been complete.

Pitfalls and Solutions

1. The incision in the lid must be angled upward, not only to avoid a through-and-through incision, but to protect the levator mechanism.

2. The most tragic complication in the patient with ectropion is caused by the failure to recognize that lid shortening has become so severe that the viability of the cornea is jeopardized by exposure and ulceration.

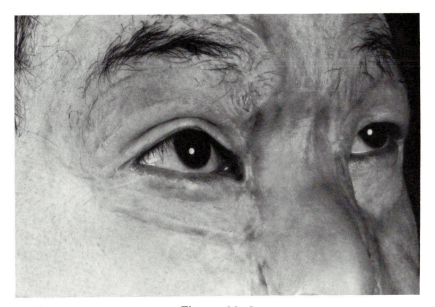

Figure 11-4

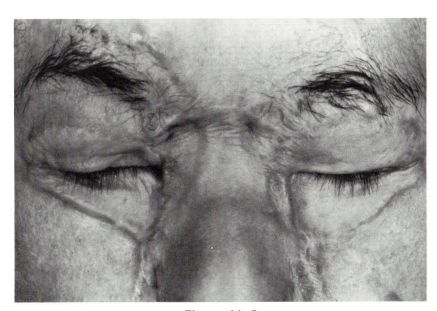

Figure 11-5

12

Lower Eyelid Ectropion

The Problem

Figure 12–1. Ectropion of the lower lid because of shortage of tissue in the vertical direction is a very common deformity. The presence of ectropion is not itself an indication for immediate surgery if there are other reconstructive priorities. Surgery should be hastened if there is chronic conjunctivitis or lack of a positive Bell's phenomenon, and danger of corneal damage. Often the upper and lower lids are involved, resulting in severe lid shortening, which forces the surgeon to operate earlier than he might wish.

Technique

Figure 12–2. Because normal anatomy is destroyed or distorted, it is wise to cannulate both lower lacrimal ducts so that the medial incision does not inadvertently damage them. The incision outlined is subciliary, and extends from the medial to the lateral canthal ligament, ending in what would be a skin crease if contracture were not present.

Figure 12–3. The incision is made to expose the orbicularis oculi muscle, and the superior flap is retracted with sutures. It is important to bevel the incision inferiorly to avoid a full-thickness cut through the conjunctiva. Note that the ends of the wound are not just small ellipses that would recontract, but that they become rectangular as the wound opens.

Figure 12–4. The graft may be partial- or full-thickness skin, and a site above the clavicle should be chosen for a good color match. The skin grafts are splinted with a tie-over dressing for seven days. Only two lids, lower or upper, are done at one time to insure that (a) the patient is able to see over the dressing and is not helpless, and (b) the defect is overcorrected rather than undercorrected. Specifically, traction on the lower lid, as seen in Figure 12–3, pulls it up over much of the upper lid, identifying a large defect. If all four lids were released only to the point at which a tarsorrhaphy could be performed, the surgeon would tend to insert smaller grafts, and early recurrence of ectropion would result.

Figure 12–5. In repose, the large skin graft not only allows for correction of the ectropion, but follows the normal curvature of the muscle and separates the lower lid from the cheek.

Pitfalls and Solutions

1. If the scalpel is not angled while the incision is made, a full-thickness cut of the conjunctiva may be made inadvertently.

2. If any distortion of the lower lid exists, the lacrimal duct should be cannulated before surgery begins.

3. Once the incision is extended to the lateral canthus, it should be continued into a "crow's-foot" to result in a full release.

LOWER EYELID ECTROPION

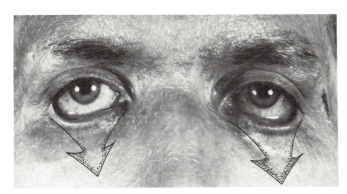
Figure 12-1

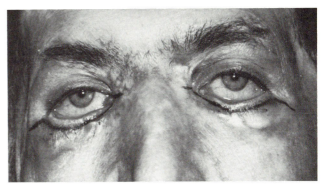
Figure 12-2

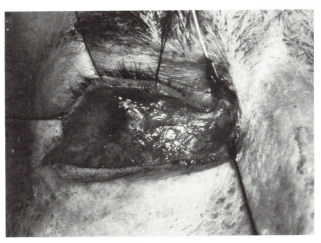
Figure 12-3

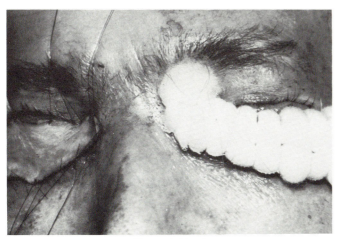
Figure 12-4

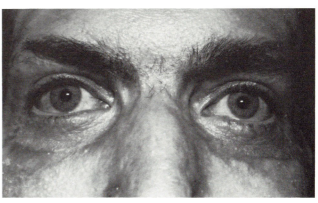
Figure 12-5

13

Resurfacing the Nose

The Problem

Full-thickness and second-degree burns of the nose may result in:

a. A patchwork appearance of grafted or spontaneously healed skin, with areas of hypertrophic scar.

b. Shortening due to alar cartilage destruction and contracture.

c. Blunting of the nasolabial angle because of scar contracture across the columella and lip.

Technique

Figures 13–1, 13–2. Areas of healed, deep, second- and third-degree burn, with previous skin graft ulcerations, have resulted in an unstable wound surface. Although the alar cartilages are intact, a burned, hypertrophic columella makes them appear retracted. The cross-hatching illustrates that all skin will be removed from the root of the nose to the tip and between both nasolabial folds. The increased nasolabial angle is due to a hypertrophic scarred columella and contracture between it and the lip.

Figure 13–3. A membranous transfixion incision was made, and an ellipse of hypertrophic scar removed from the columella in an attempt to make it less prominent. The incision was closed with sutures tied over cotton bolsters, maintaining the columella in a new position. No external release of the columella, such as a V-Y advancement, was done, because the upper lip area was to be excised and grafted as the next step in reconstruction, and further correction could be done at that time, if necessary.

Figures 13–4, 13–5. After the nose has been infiltrated with epinephrine (1:200,000) for hemostasis, dermabrasion of the dorsum is performed. Although excision is feasible, dermabrasion is a surer method to achieve a smoother surface. The sides of the nose should not be dermabraded in a straight line down the nasolabial creases, or a linear scar may result. The wounds are feathered in a Z- or S-shape.

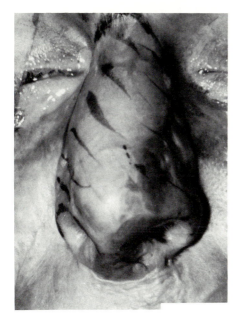

Figure 13-1

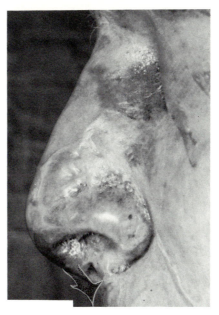

Figure 13-2

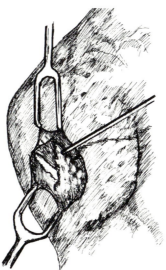

Figure 13-3

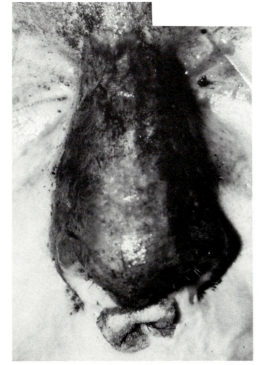

Figure 13-4

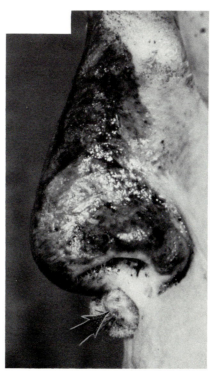

Figure 13-5

Figures 13–6, 13–7. A single split-thickness graft (0.018 to 0.020 inches thick) from a supraclavicular area such as the scalp is used for coverage. Location of the suture line is extremely important so that the nasal tip scars do not become the most prominent feature of the face. Superiorly, the suture line is between the medial canthi; laterally, it is a continuation of the nasolabial creases, but interdigitated in S- or Z-shaped incisions. Inferiorly, it is best to trace the edge of the nostril, and taper medially into the columella. A bolster dressing of foam rubber, cut to conform to the wound, is tied over the surface of the graft, and should be maintained in place for seven days.

Figures 13–8, 13–9. Six months later the corrected nose is uniform in color and texture. The nasolabial angle is no longer as obtuse, but will need further release by an external approach when the upper lip area is resurfaced.

Pitfalls and Solutions

1. When using a dermabrader at the root of the nose, the surgeon must beware of engaging the eyelashes and destroying the lid.

2. The lower lateral cartilages are superficial, and dermabrasion must be done lightly or they will be exposed.

3. In positioning the graft on the dorsum, it must be sutured over the leading edge of the alae, or a displeasing scar may result.

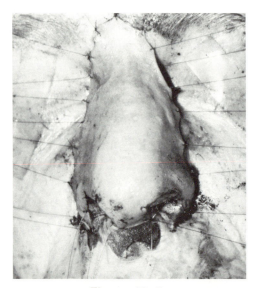

Figure 13–6

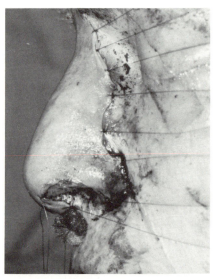

Figure 13–7

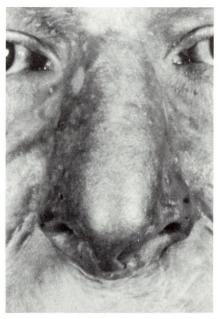

Figure 13–8

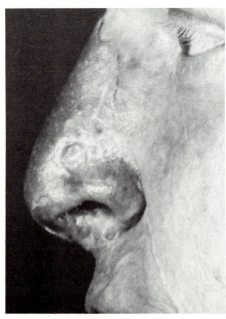

Figure 13–9

14

Radiation Injury of the Lip

The Problem

Figure 14–1. Radiation therapy of the upper lip for dermatologic problems during childhood resulted in chronic degenerative changes including:

a. Loss of substance of the lip and upper lip area. Note the lip pulled superiorly because of contracture. This is the patient's resting expression; she is not smiling.

b. Marked thinning, atrophy, and depigmentation of the tissue remaining. One notes the pale scar and irregular vermilion where Cupid's bow should be. The philosophy of reconstruction must include excision of the damaged area and replacement with surrounding normal tissue, if possible.

Technique

Figure 14–2. The area of injury to be excised is marked in a shield pattern, which will lengthen the upper lip on closure. Bilateral advancement flaps that extend around each nostril are outlined. Both the nasolabial creases and the vermilion-cutaneous border of the lip are marked to avoid any disorientation if operative edema becomes significant.

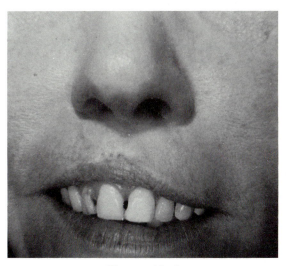

Figure 14–1

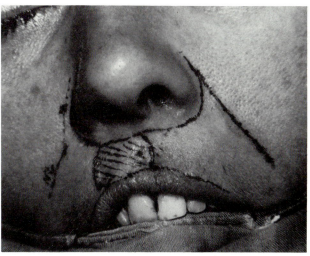

Figure 14–2

Figures 14–3, 14–4. The lesion is excised and advancement flaps cut.

Figure 14–5. A single suture through the tattooed vermilion border avoids a vermilion mismatch. A small Z-plasty is marked to prevent a straight line scar that would retract the lip.

Figure 14–6. The lip is everted to allow for closure of muscle and mucosa in separate layers. The mucosa has been cut in a Z-shape to discourage formation of a linear scar contracture.

Figure 14–7. Interrupted sutures of 6-0 monofilament in the skin, reinforced with adhesive strips, result in a reasonable scar.

Figure 14–8. Puckering of the lips reveals an intact and functioning sphincter.

Figure 14–9. In repose there is no whistle deformity or vertical scar contracture.

Pitfalls and Solutions

1. Failure to repair the orbicularis oris muscle will result in a wide scar and poor function of the lip.

2. A straight line scar will result in retraction and a whistle deformity. A Z-plasty must be incorporated into the closure, utilizing the same principles as for a cleft lip repair.

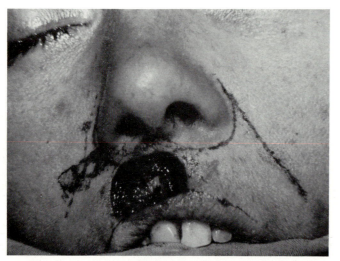

Figure 14–3

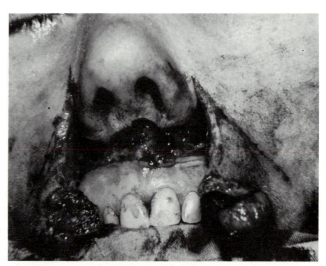

Figure 14–4

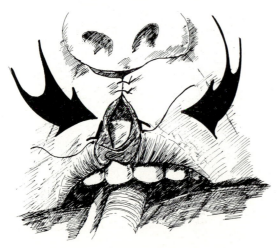

Figure 14–5

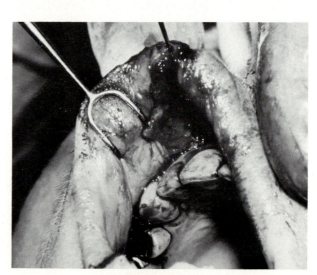

Figure 14–6

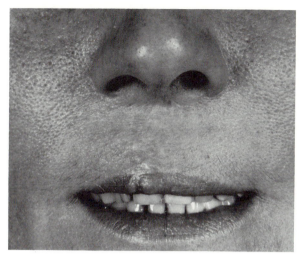

Figure 14-7

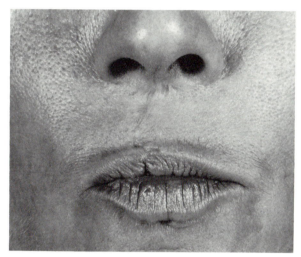

Figure 14-8

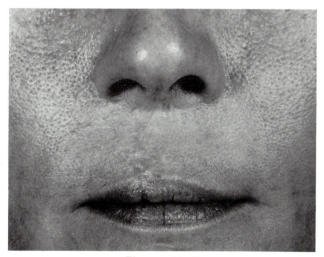

Figure 14-9

15

Reconstruction of the Oral Commissures

The Problem

Deformity of the oral commissure(s) may result from direct injury (as is often seen in children with electrical cord burns), or secondarily owing to contracture of burned perioral skin. Reconstructive methods traditionally have focused on widening the contracted oral aperture by advancing lip vermilion and oral mucosa laterally at the commissures. These procedures are frequently inadequate because:

a. There has been absolute loss of vermilion, and simply attenuating it laterally leads to recontracture;

b. The orbicularis oris muscle is often thinned or disrupted at the commissure, and is left unrepaired;

c. The commissure is displaced medially owing to vertical scarring and shortening of the perioral skin; or

d. Splinting has not been used during the healing phase, with resultant failure of remodeling of the aperture in the reconstructed, enlarged position.

Figures 15–1, 15–2. This child sustained a burn of the right oral commissure by chewing on an electrical cord. The wound healed primarily, resulting in a shortage of vermilion, linear skin contracture at the raphe, and medial displacement of the commissure due to muscle disruption and shortening. When the patient opens his mouth, the contractures are rigidly applied to the muscular raphe, limiting all movements of the lips and mouth.

Figure 15–3. The vermilion margins, peaks of the Cupid's bow, and proposed incision through the raphe of the right commissure are marked.

Figure 15–4. The incisions open the perioral tissues, leaving the medial junction of oral mucosa and vermilion intact. The damaged and scarred orbicularis oris muscle is exposed, and perioral skin has been dissected free on the subcutaneous scar.

Figure 15–5. The vermilion and intact medial commissure are retracted laterally into the soft tissue defect. The muscle is left unrepaired.

Figure 15–6. With some tension, the vermilion has been sutured to the periphery of the perioral skin incision.

Figures 15–7, 15–8. Postoperatively, there is no improvement in the resting position. The healed wound at the vermilion-skin juncture is linear and somewhat hypertrophic. When the patient opens his mouth, all the preoperative problems are still present, causing persistent deformity of the oral commissure.

Reconstruction of the oral commissure must therefore include: (a) altering vertical perioral skin contracture; (b) repair and repositioning of the orbicularis oris muscle at its raphe; (c) resurfacing of the wound defect with appropriate tissues; and (d) maintenance of the position of the mucosa, vermilion, muscle, and skin postoperatively.

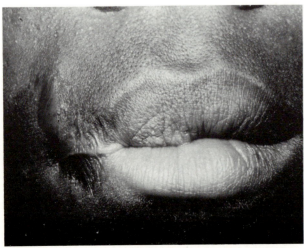

Figure 15–1

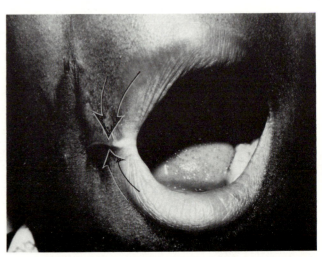

Figure 15–2

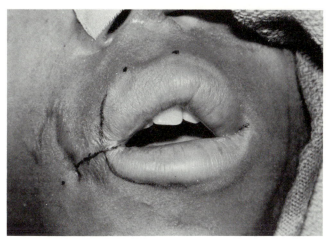

Figure 15-3

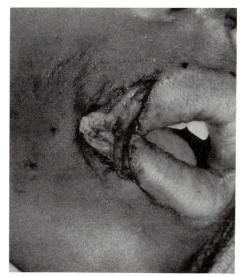

Figure 15-4

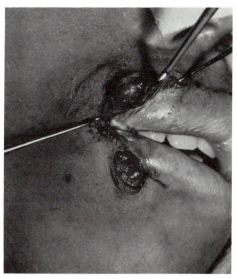

Figure 15-5

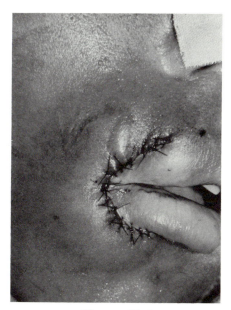

Figure 15-6

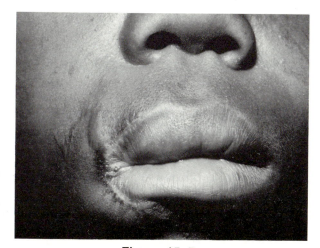

Figure 15-7

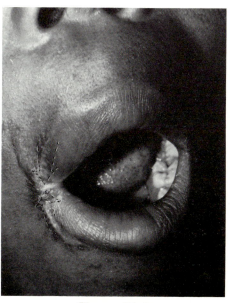

Figure 15-8

Technique

Consideration of the normal anatomy and surface appearance of the oral commissures must be taken preoperatively.

Figure 15–9. In the resting position, the lower lip skin-vermilion junction parallels that of the upper lip as they approach the commissure. Normally, more lower lip vermilion is exposed near the commissure than that of the upper lip. The upper lip slightly overlies the lower at the commissure.

Figure 15–10. In the mid-open position, the lower lip is seen to remain fuller than the upper lip at the commissure. Also, the plane of the lower lip actually is nearly perpendicular to that of the upper lip. The upper lip lies slightly anterior to the lower lip at the commissure, creating a natural overhang.

Figure 15–11. With the mouth fully open, the skin and vermilion of both lips coalesce owing to the tension of the orbicularis oris muscle itself, and the tethering effect of the other perioral muscles of facial expression. The vermilion and oral mucosa of the lower lip are still fuller than in the upper lip, and continue behind and medial to the overhang of the upper lip, into the oral cavity.

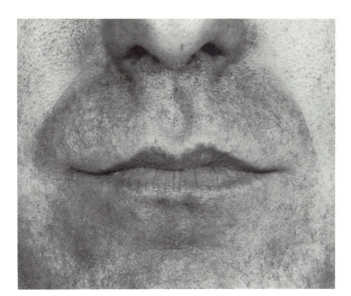
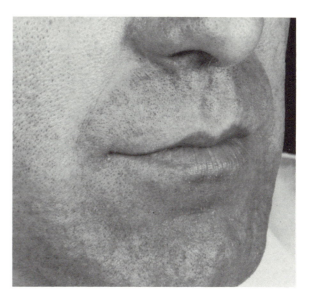

Figure 15-9

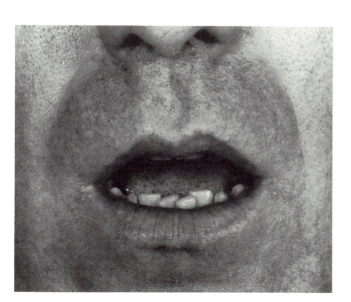
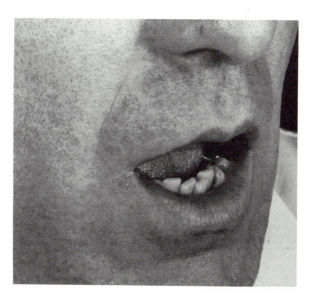

Figure 15-10

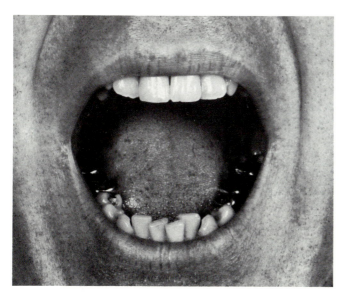
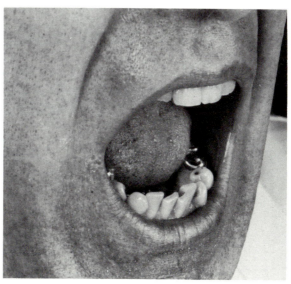

Figure 15-11

Figure 15–12. This patient sustained deep facial burns of the perioral skin and commissures, including the vermilion. There is narrowing of the oral aperture, and obliteration of the relationship of the upper and lower lips as they near the commissures.

An operative procedure based on the normal anatomical findings, as indicated, is required to correct the several abnormalities in this patient. The aperture of the mouth must be enlarged, the vertical constricting scar must be eliminated, the upper lip must be resurfaced at the lateral margins, and the lower lip must be repositioned in proper relationship to the upper lip at the commissures.

Figure 15–13. Four critical operative steps are outlined in this illustration.

A. A triangular flap of scar is elevated, with its medial limb ending at the horizontal commissure, and the incision is carried into the oral cavity at an angle similar to the lateral incision of the triangular flap. This intraoral incision is made at the inner junction of the vermilion and oral mucosa.

B. The triangular flap is retracted, and the oral mucosa previously incised is undermined and advanced to fill the defect left by the flap. At this time the fibers of the orbicularis oris muscle are dissected free superior to the horizontal raphe, and retracted inferiorly. The advanced oral mucosa is then sutured to the skin margin resulting from elevation of the retracted triangular flap of scar.

C. The triangular flap of scar is excised at its base, leaving a transverse wound extending horizontally from the oral cavity at the commissure. The muscle fibers of the orbicularis oris are then retracted *inferior* to the horizontal raphe, and are sutured to securely overlap the muscle fibers of the lower lip, and any associated fascia that is intact laterally and inferiorly. An incision is then made along the vermilion-cutaneous border of the lower lip, across the vermilion at the commissure, and posteriorly to join the previously made incision that allowed advancement of oral mucosa of the upper lip.

D. The lower lip is then advanced medially and intraorally, suturing the lateral skin to the mucosa from the upper lip in the horizontal line of the commissure. Further, the leading edge of the lower lip vermilion is sutured to the intraoral portion of upper lip mucosa at the commissure, and within the oral cavity.

Figure 15–14. At surgery, steps *A* and *B* have been carried out. On the patient's right side the advanced mucosa has been sutured, and the retracted triangular flap of skin lies loosely at the commissure. On the patient's left side the mucosa has been sutured, and the orbicularis oris muscle fibers superior to the raphe are retracted inferiorly beneath the mucosal closure.

Figure 15–15. At surgery, steps *C* and *D* have been completed. On the patient's right one can see that in fact a form of Z-plasty has been performed, except that, contrary to the usual applications of Z-plasty, the outer, or scar tissue, flap of the Z-plasty is discarded. Its wound surface has been replaced with intact, advanced, upper lip oral mucosa. Further, the lower lip has been advanced as the other flap of the Z-plasty into the oral cavity medial to the upper lip repair. The orbicularis oris muscle of the upper lip has been repositioned beneath these wounds, as previously described.

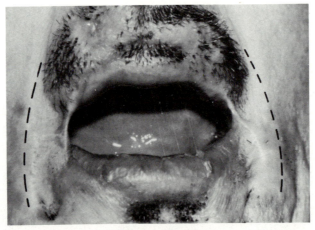

Figure 15–12

RECONSTRUCTION OF THE ORAL COMMISSURES

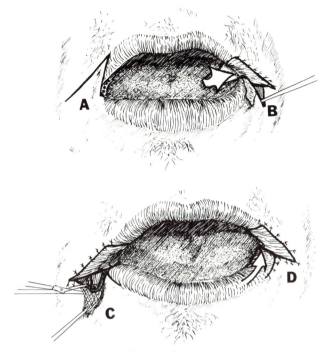

Figure 15-13

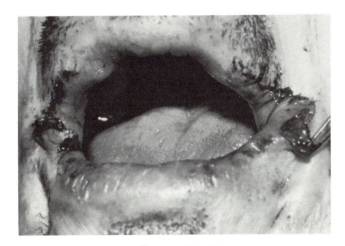

Figure 15-14

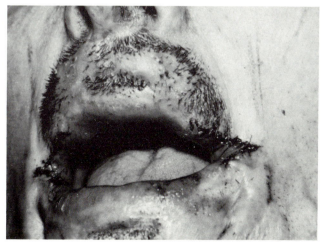

Figure 15-15

BURNS OF THE FACE

Figure 15–16. At this point, with all wounds repaired, a preformed splint is applied. In this patient, flanges made of dental acrylic material were attached to his upper dentures. These flanges are designed to lie in the horizontal plane of the oral commissures, and maintain the width of the repaired structures. If a patient does not have dentures, a partial dental plate fashioned preoperatively is used.

Figure 15–17. Several days following surgery, the patient, having worn the splint continuously except for cleansing and taking a soft diet, is shown with the splint in place. If pressure at the commissures is excessive, the flanges may be bent medially to relieve such pressure. The splint is worn for three to four weeks, as continuously as possible.

Figures 15–18, 15–19. The patient is shown three months after reconstruction of the oral commissures. In the mid-open position the lower lip is seen to lie in a nearly normal relationship with respect to the upper lip at the commissures. The commissures are continuous, with the upper lip lying slightly lateral to the lower lip, as is normally the case in this position. In the oblique view the external margin of the commissure consists only of skin, as in the normal state, with the lower lip vermilion tapering into the oral cavity beneath the overlying upper lip oral mucosa.

Figure 15–20. Eight months following surgery the configuration of the mouth is reasonable, with maintenance of the reconstructed anatomy as shown in the open-mouth view.

Pitfalls and Solutions

1. Some patients will have lesser deformities of the oral commissures, and local, definitive procedures may be adequate. If, however, there are distortions of the normal anatomy, vertical scar banding from upper to lower lip at the commissures, and medially-displaced commissures, a procedure such as suggested is warranted.

2. Splinting is critical for the maintenance of the configuration of the oral commissures after surgery.

3. Significant burns of the perioral tissues and commissures, in particular, are often deeper than initially suspected. Electrical injuries commonly are full thickness in extent. In these situations a repair that reconstructs the oral mucosa, orbicularis oris muscle, vermilion, and perioral skin is required, similar to that needed in reconstruction of a cleft lip.

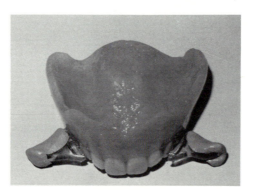

Figure 15–16

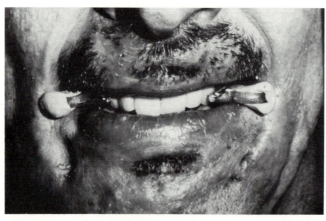

Figure 15–17

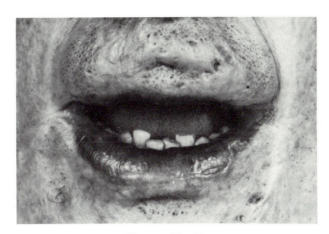

Figure 15–18

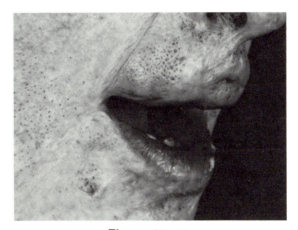

Figure 15–19

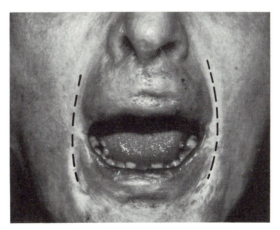

Figure 15–20

16

Perioral Hypertrophic Burn Scars: Upper Lip and Lower Lip-Chin Unit

The Problem

Perioral burn scars involving the upper lip or lower lip-chin units are esthetically and functionally disabling. Even when the whole unit is not involved, it is usually best to excise and resurface it completely. There is no excess of soft tissue in this area, and excision with primary closure of hypertrophic scars is unsightly, or ultimately distorts the lip. When the commissures are involved, there is often the additional problem of microstomia. The combined defect is very difficult to repair in one stage because postoperative immobilization of the grafts with dressings would make eating or speaking almost impossible. The patient's usual complaints are related not only to appearance, but to difficulty in attempting to open the mouth.

Technique

Figures 16-1, 16-2. In this case the patient's ability to open his mouth is limited by surrounding hypertrophic scar, but the commissures are normal. There are thus several choices available in planning the excision and coverage of the wound. In this case it was elected to correct the upper lip unit first. The juncture of the two repairs (upper and lower units) and prospective scars may be transverse or oblique at the commissures, or placed obliquely beneath them.

Figure 16-3. It is imperative to make all the skin markings before surgery to avoid the possibility of asymmetry when the patient is anesthetized and intubated. Nasal intubation for anesthesia is desirable when operating around the mouth, but it may be impossible, and the oral tube should be centered (as in cleft lip repair). The area to be excised is infiltrated with epinephrine, 1:200,000, before excision to help control troublesome bleeding. An excision is made extending obliquely below the commissures, removing the scar that restricted the mouth's being opened. Care is taken to carve the apices of the Cupid's bow in a V-shape, because the action of the orbicularis sphincter will tend to flatten it postoperatively, creating an unnatural straight line for the upper lip.

PERIORAL HYPERTROPHIC BURN SCARS: UPPER LIP AND LOWER LIP-CHIN UNIT

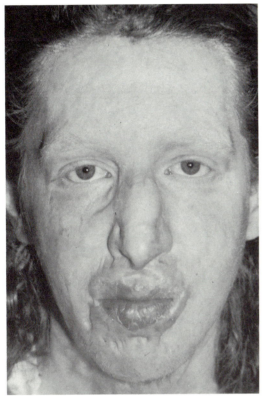

Figure 16-1

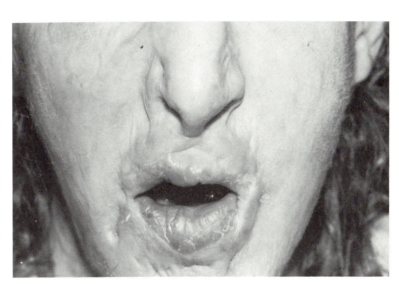

Figure 16-2

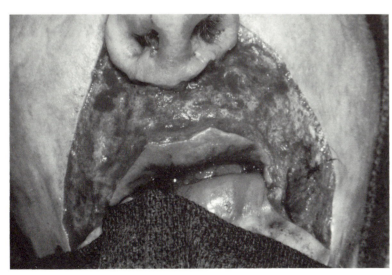

Figure 16-3

Figures 16–4, 16–5. The lower lip-chin unit was excised and grafted with scalp skin three months later, the resultant coverage being smooth, with a good color match. The donor skin is taken from the scalp or posterior neck. (Any convoluted areas of the scalp can be smoothed by subcutaneous injection of saline.) Both areas give excellent color match, can be hidden by hair, and will not result in further disfiguration. The graft (0.018 inches thick) gives satisfactory coverage, but leaves donor site hair follicles intact and does not result in hair being transplanted to the face. Six months postoperatively the patient could open his mouth widely, and there was no evidence of contracture.

Figures 16–6, 16–7. The patient also had a release and resurfacing of the neck contracture, and his total splinting regimen included:

a. An upper lip conformer with a commissure extender (Fig. 16–6).

b. A molded neck conformer (Fig. 16–7).

c. A face mask for compression of all facial scars.

Pitfalls and Solutions

1. Failure to excise the whole unit will result in a patchwork effect that is extremely distracting and offers little esthetic improvement.

2. The plane of dissection should be superficial to the orbicularis oris muscle — troublesome bleeding would result from incising or excising it.

3. The Cupid's bow should be cut in an acute V-shape to counteract the action of the orbicularis oris muscle, which tends to flatten it into a straight line.

PERIORAL HYPERTROPHIC BURN SCARS: UPPER LIP AND LOWER LIP-CHIN UNIT

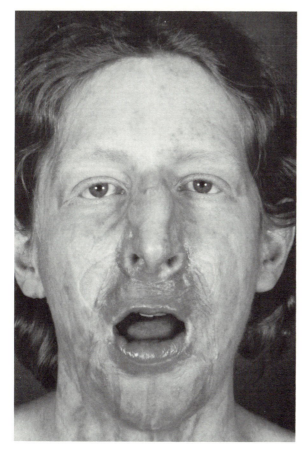

Figure 16–4

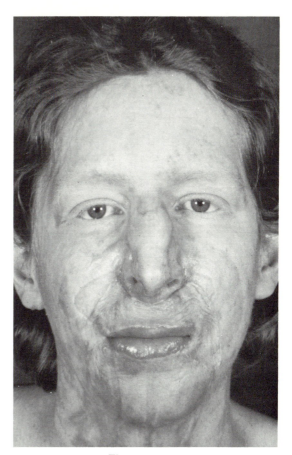

Figure 16–5

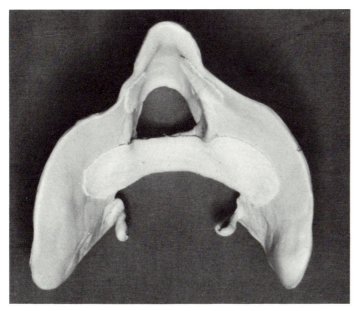

Figure 16–6

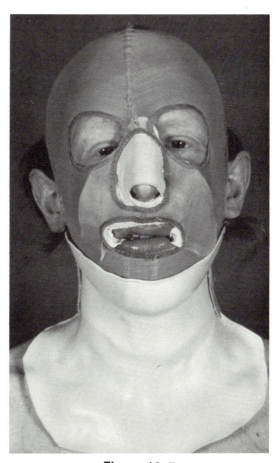

Figure 16–7

17

Reconstruction of the Lower Labial Sulcus

The Problem

Surface injury to the lips and vermilion results from many thermal burns, and injury to the labial sulcus is frequent after electrical injury in this area. Incontinence of the mouth, interference with eating, and derangements of the teeth, especially in children, are sequelae of deformity of the lower labial sulcus.

Figure 17–1. A patient is seen a few days after sustaining an electrical injury from chewing on an electrical light cord. Partial-thickness injury to the upper lip involving the vermilion was present, but the severe portion of the injury was through the full thickness of the lower lip, with obliteration of the labial sulcus. It is important to maintain the dimensions of the oral aperture in this situation. Early excision of this area should not be done because the final result is often one of vermilion mismatch, foreshortening of the length of the lip, and contracture of the lateral dimension of the lower lip due to overestimation of the injury at the time of early resection.

It is preferable to construct an oral appliance to be used as soon after the injury as possible. Orthodontic or prosthdontic consultation is required in most instances.

Figure 17–2. An acrylic splint is applied, fitted to the oral aperture, and designed with lateral wings abutting on the oral commissures. The splint is worn continuously except during eating and maintenance of oral hygiene. In the initial several days the splint is removed frequently to observe any lateral ulceration caused by pressure, and to adjust it accordingly.

Figure 17–3. After seven days of treatment the oral aperture is being maintained, and there is gradual surface healing of the wound.

Figure 17–4. At five weeks from injury the upper lip has healed well, and the lower lip has healed with a small, hypertrophic scar. The dimensions of the oral aperture have been maintained adequately.

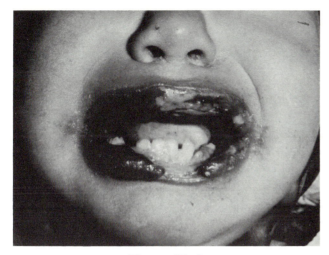

Figure 17-1

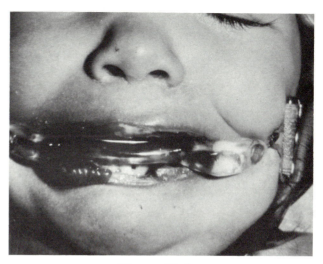

Figure 17-2

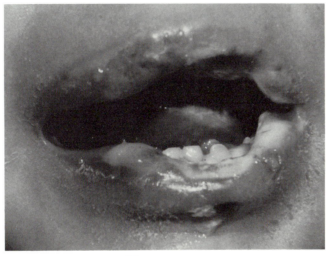

Figure 17-3

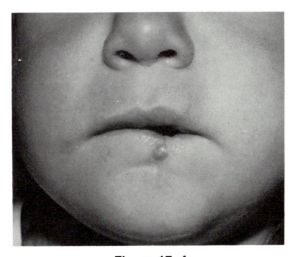

Figure 17-4

Figure 17–5. There is obliteration of the lower labial sulcus, and a synechia between the mucosa of the lower lip and the anterior gingiva, extending to the alveolar ridge.

Figure 17–6. Incision and recreation of the full extent of the lower labial sulcus is done, three months after the initial injury. The incision is made at the upper margin of the contracted wound, near the alveolar margin. Dissection is carried out inferiorly and deeply, separating the mucosa that remains on the upper, inner aspect of the lower lip from the gingival mucosa.

Figure 17–7. In cross-section the recreation of the lower labial sulcus is illustrated.

Figure 17–8. At this point a moulage is made, using rapid-curing, acrylic dental compound. The dental material is molded into place so that the sulcus is defined, not only in its lateral extent, but vertically, to the level of the intact gingiva internally, and the intact lip mucosa externally. The dental material is placed over the lower teeth to provide later stability.

The prepared moulage is seen from its inner surface. The upper lateral extensions will lie over the teeth, providing stability during the healing process. A drill hole is placed through the lower portion of the moulage to allow passage of a 4-0 monofilament suture through the alveolar ridge below, upward, and over it, between two adjacent teeth. This suture is tied at the completion of the procedure to maintain the position of the moulage.

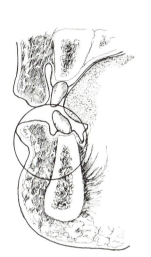

Figure 17-5

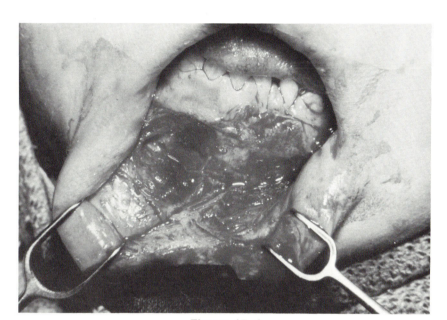

Figure 17-6

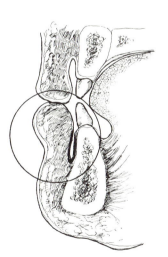

Figure 17-7

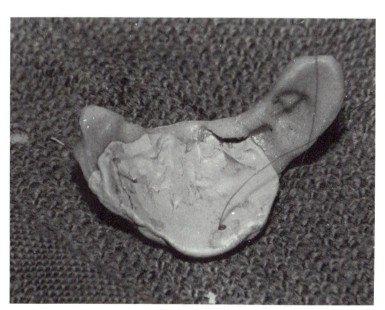

Figure 17-8

Figures 17–9, 17–10. A medium-thickness (0.014- to 0.016-inch) skin graft is sutured into place over the gingival surface of the defect with 5-0 synthetic, absorbable material. The remainder of the skin graft lies at the depth of the labial sulcus, and is brought upward to resurface the labial mucosal defect. The previously prepared moulage is then placed into position over the gingival skin graft. The 4-0 monofilament suture is passed through the alveolus, upward behind it, and forward between two incisors. It is tied to the end of the suture protruding from the drill hole in the moulage. This will anchor the moulage in the lower labial sulcus.

The moulage splint is maintained in place for approximately two weeks. Frequent inspection of the operative site and the position of the moulage is necessary for wound cleansing and assessment of graft healing. A largely liquid diet is prescribed during the period of early healing. Following removal of the moulage, a soft, nonchewing diet is continued for three weeks. During this time the mouth is washed with water after each meal, to prevent retention of food material in the labial sulcus.

Figures 17–11, 17–12. The patient is shown several months following reconstructive surgery. The lower labial sulcus is restored.

Pitfalls and Solutions

1. Early excision of this type of wound of the lip and labial sulcus should be avoided. Maintenance of the oral aperture is best accomplished by means of splinting until healing and remodeling of the tissues is achieved.

2. Simultaneous resection or revision of associated lip scars and defects is often required. Marking of the vermilion-cutaneous junctions will avoid mismatching these structures during repair, and consequent creation of a "stair-step" deformity.

3. If concomitant repair of a lip defect is done, skin, muscle, and mucosal layers are repaired individually to insure full function and appearance of the resulting lip.

4. Orthodontic or prosthodontic consultation may be needed for proper selection of materials, and appropriate placement of the splint and moulage over the lower teeth and in the lower labial sulcus.

RECONSTRUCTION OF THE LOWER LABIAL SULCUS

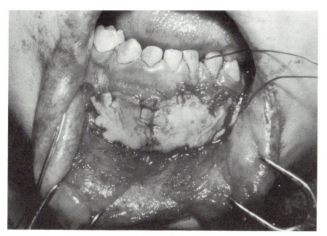

Figure 17-9

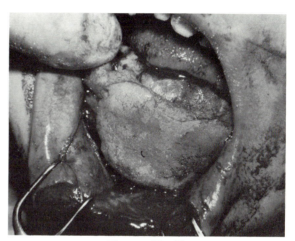

Figure 17-10

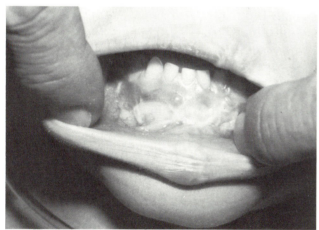

Figure 17-11

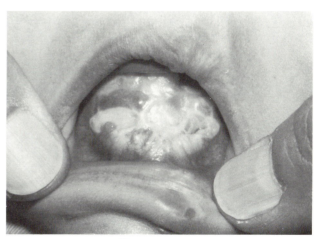

Figure 17-12

18

The Everted Lower Lip

The Problem

The effect of a healed burn of the chin, lower lip, and vermilion is to produce a consolidation of these areas into a mass, with eversion of the lower lip and vermilion. Traditional methods of skin grafting, without particular emphasis on the underlying anatomy of these areas and their relationship to one another as portions of facial units, may lead to a recurrence of scarring and deformity. Because of the vulnerability of the vermilion and lower lip to deformity after burn injury and simple skin grafting, carefully planned splinting is also required. All contours of the vermilion and lower lip-chin facial unit, with separation from the upper neck, are otherwise lost.

Figures 18-1, 18-2. This patient had excision of a deep burn of the lower lip and chin, and application of thin (0.010-inch) skin grafts with no external support of the lower facial structures. The vermilion and oral mucosa became everted. After several months these tissues were attenuated and often excoriated, and the grafts over the lower lip developed hypertrophic scarring.

Technique

Figure 18-3. An area of chronically exposed and scarred vermilion is marked for excision. Superiorly, the mucosa of the lower lip has become everted. Inferior to the shaded area of vermilion, the entire lower lip sulcus and surrounding region consists of hypertrophic scar.

Figure 18-4. The incision and dissection through scar, to expose and completely release the stretched orbicularis oris muscle over its length from one commissure to the other, is illustrated. This muscle had become markedly attenuated and unsupportive of the lower lip because of the contracture from below.

Figure 18-5. Excision of the chronically damaged vermilion is done. The lower lip-chin angle is re-created by excision of the scar to the level of the orbicularis oris muscle. If necessary, the slinglike orbicularis oris muscle is undermined along its length to allow complete upward mobility.

Figure 18-6. A skin graft of medium thickness (0.016 inches) taken from the scalp is applied to the lower lip sulcus. The graft is sutured into position with 5-0 monofilament material, with the suture ends left long. A nonadherent gauze dressing is applied and covered with a soft, occlusive gauze bolster, which is held in place by tying the long ends of the sutures over it.

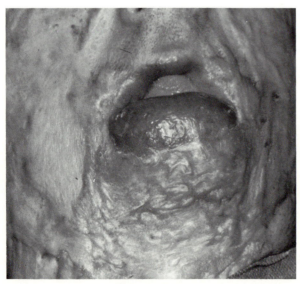

Figure 18-1

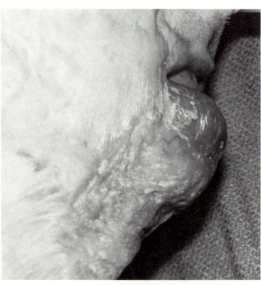

Figure 18-2

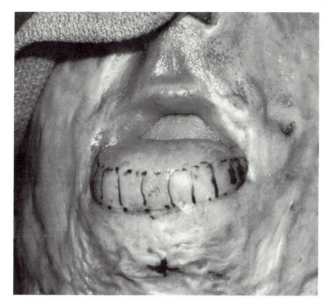

Figure 18-3

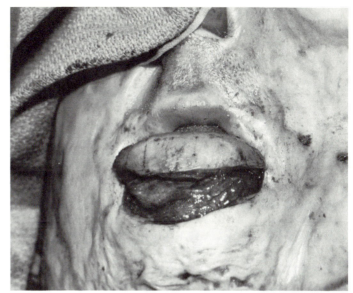

Figure 18-4

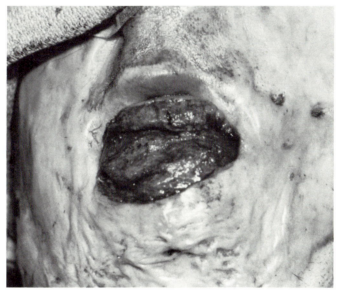

Figure 18-5

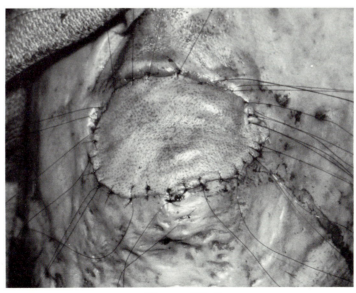

Figure 18-6

Figure 18–7, 18–8. After an initial period of skin graft healing, usually seven days, the dressings are removed and a specially designed splint is applied. The splint consists of two important components:

(a) A lower, submental portion that maintains pressure and definition of the mental prominence with respect to the upper neck. This portion will also support the chin by means of upward force, maintaining the cervicomental angle.

(b) A removable, transverse component that applies pressure and support to define the lower lip-chin angle. This portion of the splint maintains upward force on the lower lip, and lies inferior to the level of the repositioned orbicularis oris muscle.

Both splints are constructed of heat-labile plastic material, fitted carefully to the individual patient. The plastic components are lined with a layer of fine, closed-cell, plastic foam, and are fitted with Velcro patches at their lateral margins so that they may be removed easily. Initially the components are removed several times daily for inspection of the graft, and so that any minor adjustments may be made to avoid pressure ulceration. The transverse portion is worn continuously, except during inspection periods, eating, and maintenance of oral hygiene. This splint must be worn for a period of at least nine months, and its importance must be emphasized frequently to the patient.

Figures 18–9, 18–10. The patient is shown early after surgery and treatment with the splinting devices. There is enhanced definition of the cervicomental and lower lip-chin angles.

Figure 18–11. Nine months following surgery and splinting, the mental prominence is recreated with a reasonable lower lip-chin angle, and separation of the contours of the lip, chin, and upper neck.

Pitfalls and Solutions

1. Complete dissection and release of the orbicularis oris muscle must be achieved at the time of surgery. If this is not done, the often atonic muscle will remain in an inferior position, and eversion of the lower lip with obliteration of the lip-chin angle will occur.

2. Frequent removal of the splints is required for inspection of the underlying tissues. Pressure ulceration will develop rapidly unless minor adjustments are made during the healing process.

3. Both preoperatively and throughout the treatment course, the patient must be apprised of the importance of wearing the splints continuously except during the times noted. Reinforcement of this concept is required, but when the patient sees the improved result he usually continues to accept the regimen.

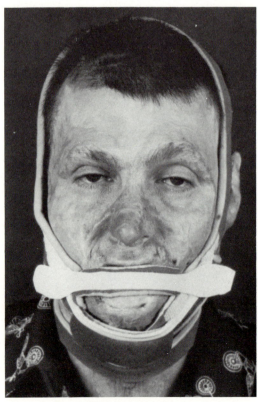

Figure 18–7

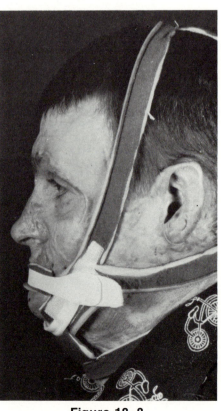

Figure 18–8

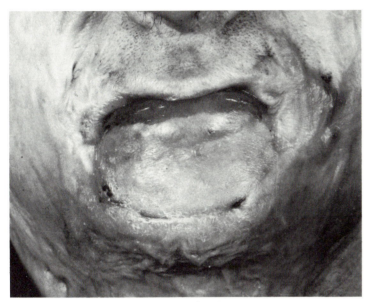

Figure 18-9

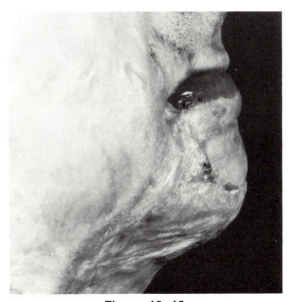

Figure 18-10

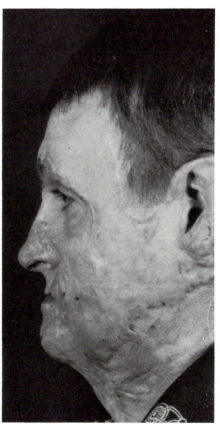

Figure 18-11

19

Lower Lip-Chin Esthetic Facial Unit

The Problem

A burn of the lower lip-chin esthetic unit may involve:

 a. The lower lip, causing eversion.
 b. Commissures of the mouth, a vertical scar band limiting the ability to open widely.
 c. Obliteration of the sulcus between the lower lip and the chin.
 d. Obliteration of the neck-chin junction.

Depending on the extent of the pathologic condition, it may be impossible to correct all these problems at one operation.

Technique

Figure 19-1. This case illustrates all the above problems, and incisions are outlined parallel to the nasolabial creases for a symmetrical effect. Superiorly, the incision follows the vermilion of the lower lip, and inferiorly, the edge of the hypertrophic scar of the neck. The contractures of the commissures will be released by transverse incisions across the constricting, hypertrophic horizontal scar.

Figure 19-2. The defect created is large, and bleeding may be a problem. It is helpful to inject the prospective site of excision with epinephrine, 1:200,000, prior to excision. Although there is a fairly avascular plane in the neck at the level of the superficial fascia, there is none in the chin below the scar, and the surgeon must be diligent in achieving hemostasis. The incision at the vermilion border of the lower lip extends to the orbicularis oris, and that muscle is released from the overlying scar throughout its entire length.

Figure 19-3. In such a large defect it is common to need more than one split-thickness graft (0.018 to 0.021 inches), and these may be joined obliquely or transversely. The suture lines should be below the border of the mandible.

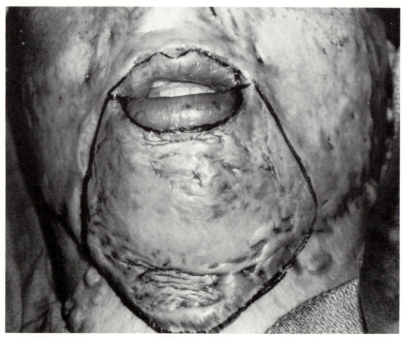

Figure 19-1

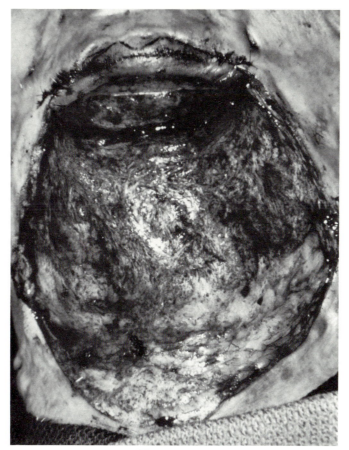

Figure 19-2

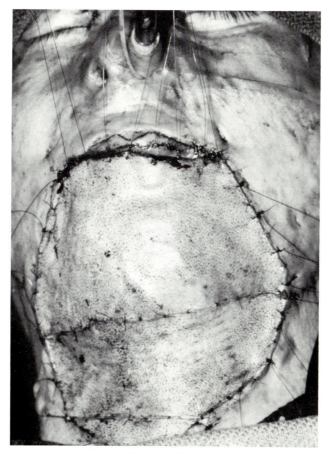

Figure 19-3

Figure 19-4. The graft is bolstered into place with a tie-over dressing of foam rubber. When the dressing is removed seven days later, the postoperative splint is crucial. If the patient refuses to wear one, he will recontract in weeks. Since all facial splints are highly visible, the patient should be shown pictures of others in the splint, or even a sample of the splint itself, before surgery is begun. If he is not prepared to wear it, and to accept his role in insuring success, the operation should not be performed. The splint must: (a) support the lower lip with pressure, as the muscle sphincter may have lost its tone from being in the contracted, everted position; and (b) separate the chin from the neck by maintaining extension. This heat-labile splint, held in place with straps, is light and performs these functions.

Figure 19-5. The smooth esthetic unit has been achieved with a narrower lower lip.

Figure 19-6. This effect may be compared with the upper lip unit, which has not yet been reconstructed and is extremely distracting, drawing the viewer's attention to this portion of the face.

Pitfalls and Solutions

1. The excised wound is very uneven and convoluted. Hemostasis must be perfect and the dressing applied meticulously, or hematoma will result.

2. The incision along the vermilion must extend to the orbicularis oris and then angle inferiorly, or the muscle will be inadvertently separated from the lip.

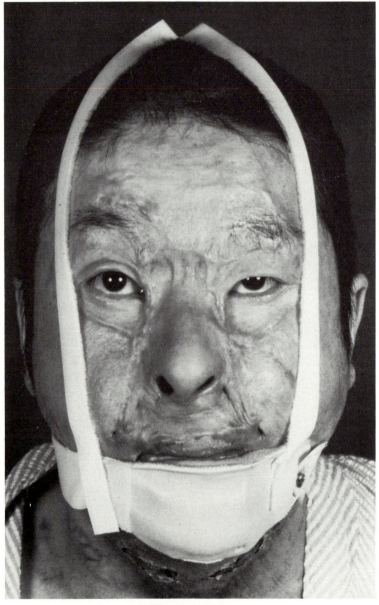

Figure 19-4

LOWER LIP-CHIN ESTHETIC FACIAL UNIT

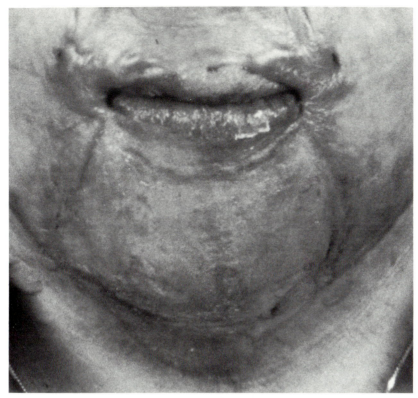

Figure 19-5

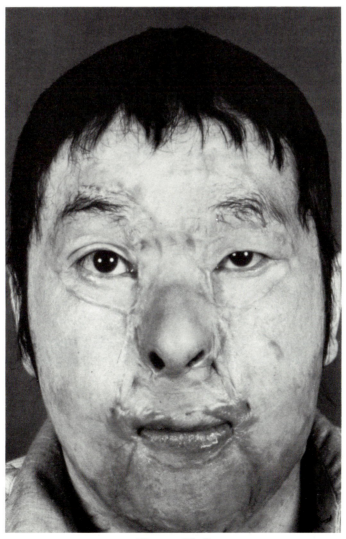

Figure 19-6

83

20

Re-creation of the Anatomical Angles of the Lower Facial Unit

The Problem

Deformity of the lower facial esthetic unit (lip-chin) is very visible for two reasons:

a. It cannot be camouflaged with hair, as with defects of the forehead, ears, and cheeks.

b. The unit is the most animated part of the face, and scarring around the mouth produces a wooden expression regardless of the patient's mood or state of mind.

Figure 20-1. The child is attempting to smile, but constricting scar limits facial expression.

Figure 20-2. Comparing the lateral and frontal views, one sees that the normal planes of the face are blunted by scar contracture. In repose, the mental prominence is lost because of lip eversion and scar that obliterates the lip-chin angle. The chin-neck juncture is a simple straight line. Placement of the skin graft juncture in the midneck, which healed with a hypertrophic scar, gives the illusion of a depressed mandibular margin.

Figure 20-3A, B. Artistic photographic license is used to illustrate the point. If one shades out the lower esthetic unit, one sees that the eyes are quite animated, as might be expected of a 13-year-old boy. When the eyes are shaded out, the abnormal lower esthetic unit is featured, revealing the loss of normal tissue planes. Thus, the problem is shortage of tissue, with scar that has destroyed or blunted the normal angles of the face in repose, severely limiting animation.

RE-CREATION OF THE ANATOMICAL ANGLES OF THE LOWER FACIAL UNIT

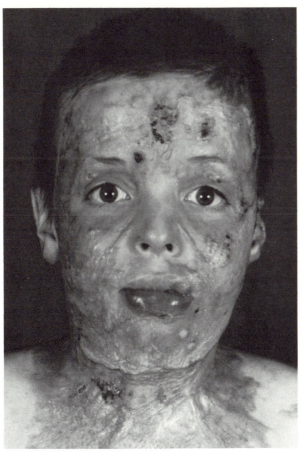

Figure 20-1

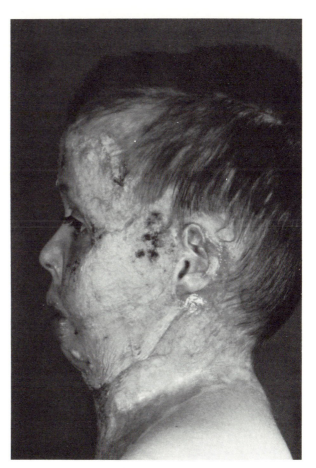

Figure 20-2

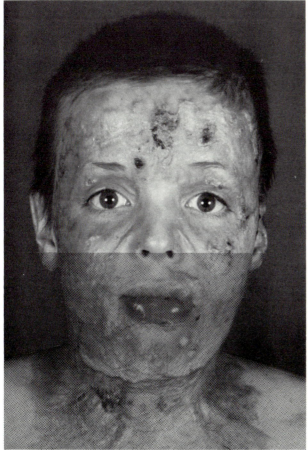

Figure 20-3A

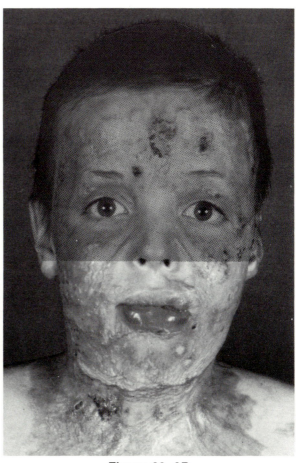

Figure 20-3B

Techniques

The treatment plan included:
 a. Surgery, to supply adequate soft tissue.
 b. Splinting — a compression garment and splints to mold normal tissue planes.

The individual techniques have been illustrated in other sections and included:
 a. Excision of the chin unit and replacement with a scalp graft.
 b. Incision of the neck contracture and excision of the hypertrophic scar; insertion of skin grafts from the scalp, with a suture line parallel to the ultimate mandibular angle.
 c. Z-plasty releases of the commissures of the mouth.

Figures 20–4, 20–5. The compression mask, if worn continuously for one year, tends to flatten the healed graft, and the new scar assumes a more uniform appearance. The heat-labile, plastic neck splint not only extends the neck, but is molded to form a new line of the mandible. Thus, the neck-chin angle will be improved. A conventional neck splint, however, will not improve the labiomental angle. Lining the superior portion of the inside of the splint with foam rubber will indent the soft tissue between the lip and chin, and support the lower lip, which is often atonic from a chronically stretched sphincter.

Figures 20–6, 20–7. The result in a full-face view reveals an animated smile. Note the clean demarcation of the chin line, the roundness of the orbicularis sphincter, and the vertical laugh-lines parallel to the chin. The lateral view reveals a clearly defined chin, with reconstituted cervicomental and lower lip-chin angles.

Pitfalls and Solutions

1. This postoperative splinting program requires frequent modification because tissue maturation proceeds over a long period. It is mandatory that the splints and garments be altered and renewed as often as necessary. To achieve the desired result, the surgeon himself should evaluate the patient frequently and direct these changes.

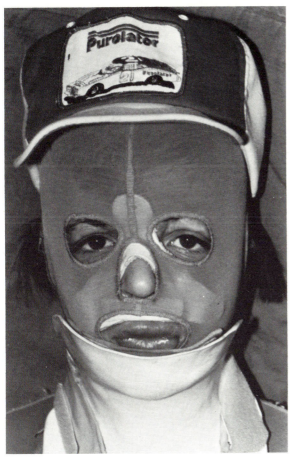
Figure 20-4

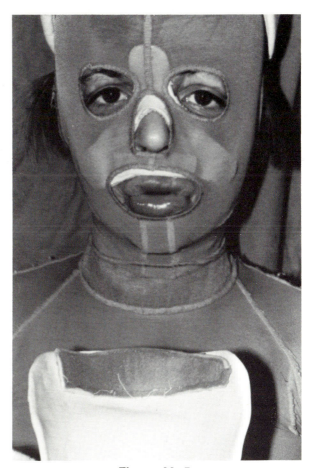
Figure 20-5

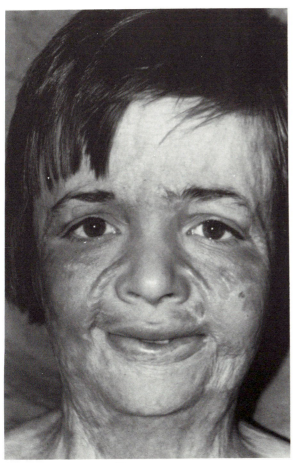
Figure 20-6

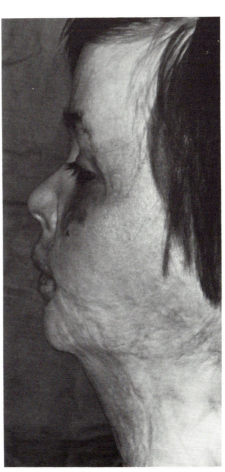
Figure 20-7

Burn Contractures of the Neck

Burn contractures of the neck are common, and become significant to patient and surgeon because of potential interference with access to the upper airway required for operative procedures. Further, they produce obvious deformity, and can limit motion of the neck and lower jaw during eating and speech. When this is associated with scarring of the lower face, the patient may have an incontinent mouth.

Contractures of the neck region may be generally grouped as follows:
a. Lateral cervical contracture.
b. Posterior, or nuchal, contracture.
c. Contracture at or above the level of the hyoid bone.
d. Contracture below the level of the hyoid.
e. Contracture involving the entire anterior surface of the neck.

Lateral and posterior contractures are very uncommon. When localized, lateral contractures in the cervical region may be treated with Z-plasty, or, if more extensive and hypertrophic, excision with skin graft coverage. Posterior contracture is usually due to hypertrophic scar, often worsened by folliculitis if the lower scalp is involved. It is best treated by excision of the scarred area and resurfacing with split-thickness skin grafts.

Preoperative consultation with an anesthesiologist is advised for all of the anterior cervical contractures, particularly if marked, with severe flexion of the neck, or when the anterior neck is covered with thickened scar. Endotracheal intubation may be impossible, and this must be anticipated before reconstructive surgery. In some severe cases the initial release of restricting scar must be done with local anesthesia, or intravenous analgesia, followed by endotracheal intubation for completion of the procedure. Many of the resulting excisional and incisional wounds are extremely hemorrhagic, and preoperative arrangements for blood replacement are mandatory.

Recently, large, local cutaneous and myocutaneous pedicle flaps have been used in selected cases for resurfacing the neck. Free myocutaneous flaps from distant donor sites, revascularized using microsurgical techniques with recipient arteriovenous channels in the cervical region, have also been used in a few patients. The results have been dramatic in terms of the resurfacing itself, but often the contour and mobility of the new tissues have not been satisfactory. These methods are useful in those patients with extraordinarily deep scar and tissue loss, and after refinement of the techniques will have a significant role in reconstruction of cervical and other defects.

21

Cervical Contracture At or Above the Level of the Hyoid

The Problem

When contracture due to scar is primarily concentrated at, or just above, the level of the hyoid bone, initial incision is best made at the hyoid level.

Figure 21–1. This situation is illustrated diagrammatically, showing the contractile forces from above (*a*) and below (*c*) acting upon the anterior neck at level *B, near the level of the hyoid.

Technique

Figures 21–2, 21–3. A patient is shown with mild contracture of the anterior neck and blunting of the cervicomental prominence. The scar in this patient was not hypertrophic, so that excision of this tissue was not required.

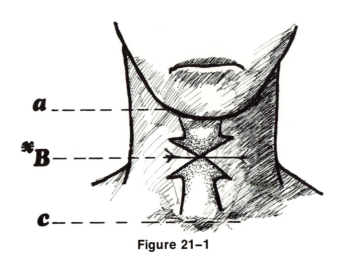

Figure 21–1

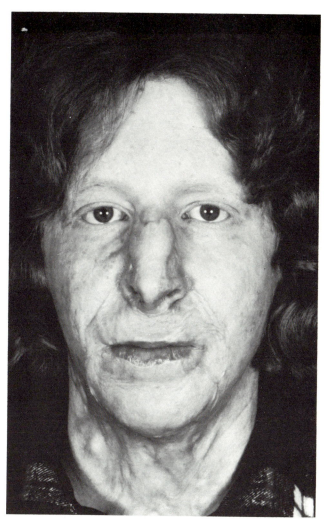

Figure 21-2

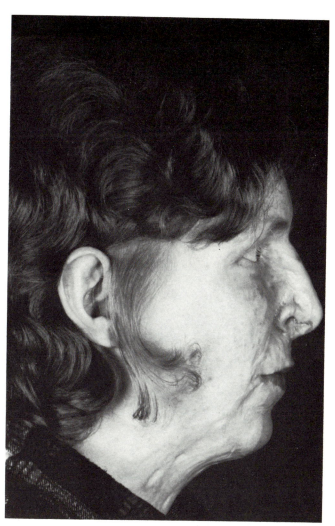

Figure 21-3

BURN CONTRACTURES OF THE NECK

Figure 21-4. A transverse incision is made at the hyoid level, so that the lateral margins lie posterior to the midlateral line of the neck on either side. Incisions that are shorter than this usually do not allow full release of the contracture, and result in less than full, passive extension of the neck. At both lateral margins, short incisions are made, radiating upward and downward at an angle of 45 degrees. This will avoid a straight, vertical incision line at the lateral margins, which often leads to local contracture and hypertrophic scarring in this area.

Figure 21-5. The dissection releases the adjacent tissues upward and downward. Dissection must be carried out in the deepest plane that is uninvolved with scar. Sometimes this plan will actually lie beneath the anterior cervical "strap" muscles in the event of very deep burn injuries. Any scarred musculature must be divided so that full, passive range of neck motion is achieved at surgery. Complete hemostasis must be accomplished by means of pressure, electrocoagulation of vessels, and repeated assessment of the operative field during the dissection. If absolute hemostasis is in doubt after completion of full release of the neck, the wound should be covered with a nonadherent, occlusive dressing, and resurfacing delayed for 24 to 48 hours. Usually, with diligent efforts using the methods cited, hemostasis and resurfacing can be done in one operative procedure.

A medium-thickness (0.016-inch) split skin graft is taken, preferably in one large sheet. The scalp is an excellent donor site for this graft because of its natural color match with facial and cervical skin. The graft is sutured into place with interrupted 5-0 monofilament material, and suture ends are left long.

Figure 21-6. A dressing composed of a nonadherent gauze layer adjacent to the skin graft and a central, bulky, absorbent layer is applied; the long, uncut ends of the sutures are tied over to provide a supportive bolster for the wound. Additional gauze padding is applied to the entire surrounding area, over which is fashioned a heat-labile plastic splint that remains in place for five to seven days during the initial healing of the skin graft.

Following healing of the graft, another cervical splint is designed with similar material, and padded with an inner layer of closed-cell foam material, 0.25 inches thick. This splint is worn by the patient as continuously as possible for from four to six months, to ensure full maintenance of neck extension. After two to three weeks, periods of splint removal are allowed for range of motion exercises.

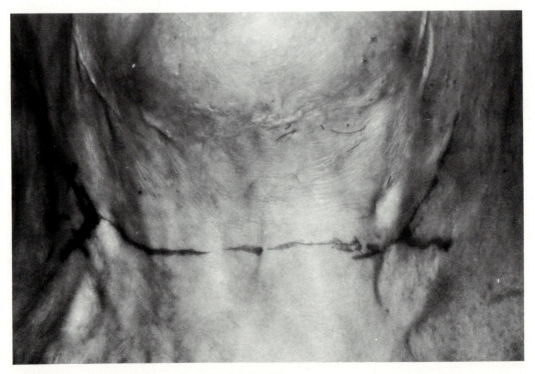

Figure 21-4

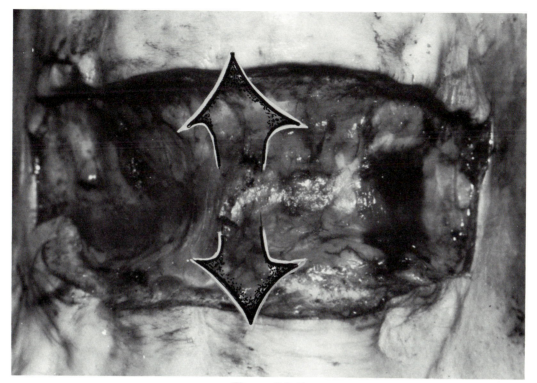

Figure 21-5

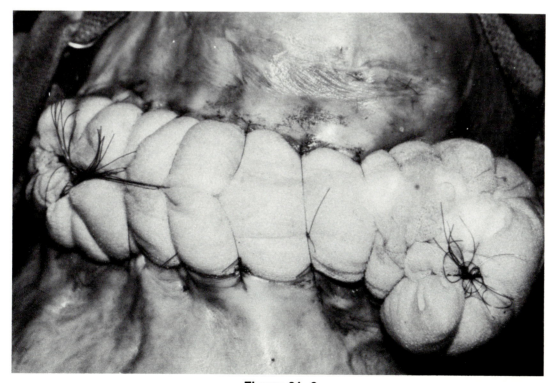

Figure 21-6

BURN CONTRACTURES OF THE NECK

Figures 21-7, 21-8. The patient is seen one year after release and resurfacing of the anterior neck.

Pitfalls and Solutions

1. Hemostasis must be complete at the initial operation or delayed resurfacing will be required. Hematoma beneath a skin graft in this area will lead to necrosis of the graft, and occasionally cause respiratory embarrassment.

2. Postoperative splinting is required to guarantee full range of motion of the neck. This fact must be emphasized repeatedly to the patient, to ensure his compliance with a long period of immobilization and intermittent exercise.

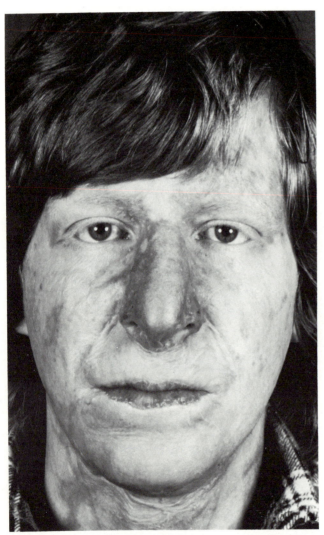

Figure 21-7

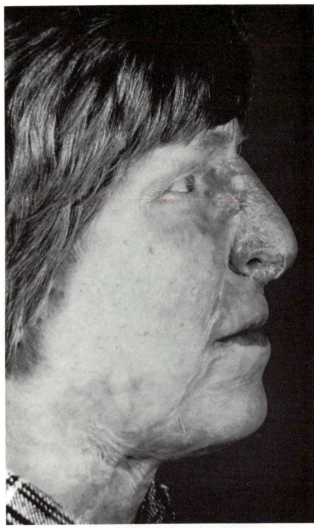

Figure 21-8

22

Cervical Contracture or Scarring Involving the Entire Anterior Surface of the Neck

The Problem

When burn contracture has involved all levels of the anterior neck, the quality of the resulting surface tissue will determine the method required for reconstruction. Massive contracture, or marked hypertrophy of the scarred tissues over the anterior neck, may result in severe deformity that is functionally and esthetically intolerable.

Technique

Figures 22–1, 22–2, 22–3. A patient is demonstrated with marked hypertrophic scarring of the anterior cervical region. In these views, the patient is attempting to extend his neck. Although the flexion contracture is not severe, the hypertrophic tissues were chronically ulcerated and esthetically poor. Incision at one level alone would not result in acceptable adjacent tissue for skin grafting and adequate release of this contracture. When possible, incision in the upper neck should not be carried on to the facial skin units. In this patient, however, the hypertrophic scar extended rather high on the cheeks, was irregular and thickened, and was therefore excised. The entire plaquelike area of scar outlined was excised.

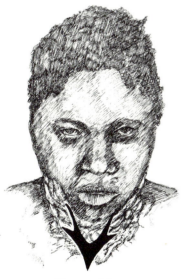

Figure 22-1

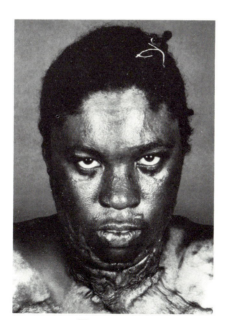

Figure 22-2

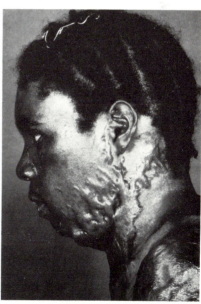

Figure 22-3

Figure 22–4. The operative wound is seen after excision of the hypertrophic scar. These excisional wounds can be of impressive surface area when release is completed, and blood loss may reach several hundred cubic centimeters. This must be anticipated in the preoperative evaluation of the patient, particularly one in the pediatric age-group. Provisions for blood replacement, adequate skin graft donor sites, and postoperative management of these large grafted surfaces must be taken into consideration prior to surgery.

Figure 22–5. The surface area of the resected specimens of hypertrophic scar is only a fraction of that of the resulting wound.

Figure 22–6. The general plan for resurfacing, using split-thickness skin grafts, is shown. Sheet grafts of maximal size are taken so that vertical junctures are avoided. Medium-thickness (0.012- to 0.016-inch) skin grafts are obtained with an electrical or air-driven dermatome so that long sheets are available, placing the junctures of the grafts transversely. The grafts are sutured into position with 5-0 monofilament material. Wounds of this dimension over the entire neck are not suitable for tie-over or bolstered dressings. A nonadherent gauze layer is applied to the sutured skin grafts, followed by a large, occlusive, absorbent dressing placed circumferentially about the neck, which is held in extension. Careful extubation in the operating room is carried out by the anesthesiologist, and assessment of the airway function is made at that time, before the patient is transported to the recovery area. Occasionally the dressing must be adjusted, or reintubation of the patient for several hours is required.

Figures 22–7, 22–8. Several months following surgery, the patient has excellent extension of the neck. Further revision of the upper thoracic area was planned to fully reconstruct the anterior cervical and thoracic regions.

Figure 22–9. A heat-labile, plastic splint is demonstrated, which is worn by the patient continuously after the initial healing of the skin grafts, except during meals and exercise periods. Whereas splinting may be required for only four to six months in lesser cervical contractures that have been resurfaced, patients with repair of the entire anterior neck region must maintain this type of splinting program for nine months to one year.

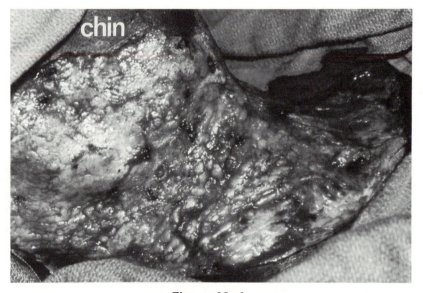

Figure 22–4

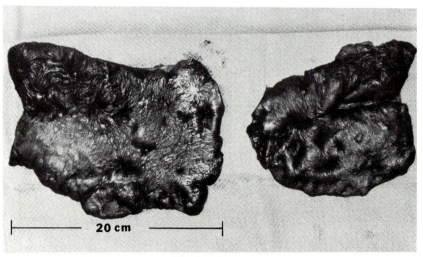

Figure 22–5

CERVICAL CONTRACTURE INVOLVING THE ENTIRE ANTERIOR SURFACE OF THE NECK

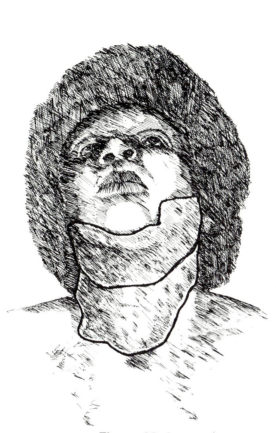

Figure 22-6

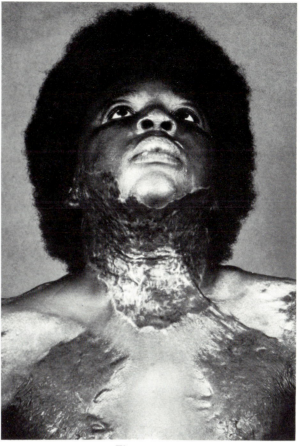

Figure 22-7

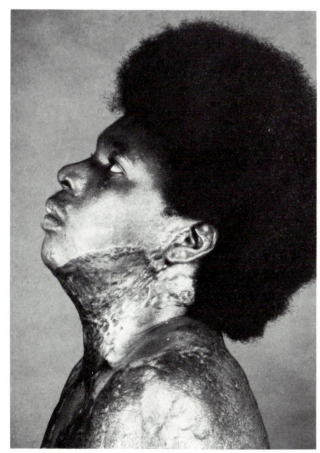

Figure 22-8

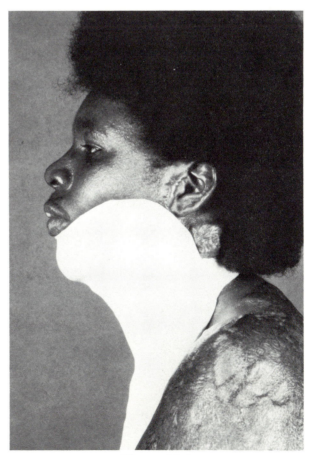

Figure 22-9

BURN CONTRACTURES OF THE NECK

Figures 22-10, 22-11. A massive contracture of the anterior neck occurred in a young girl. Fortunately, with current early management techniques, this type of deformity is avoidable today. The lower lip vermilion is everted and is adherent to the tissues over the upper thorax, resulting in pronounced downward distraction of the lower face, incontinence of the mouth, and total restriction of head movement. Consultation with the anesthesiologist was obtained to anticipate airway accessibility, and plan for partial release of the contracture with local anesthesia, followed by endotracheal intubation.

Figure 22-12. The levels for incision at *A and *C are illustrated. The skin of most of the lower face was uninvolved with scarring, so that incision at *A would allow upward displacement of the face when separated from the lower contracture. Whenever possible, incisions above the mandibular margin should be avoided because of encroachment upon the confines of the facial esthetic units, which result in unsatisfactory scar lines. With intravenous analgesia and local anesthesia, enough release was achieved so that endotracheal intubation was accomplished and the dissection could be continued. This dissection is done in the deepest plane that is not involved with scar. In this case, some of the anterior cervical musculature was divided. The level of the hyoid is at *b*. The lower incision is made at the cervicothoracic junction, *C. Laterally, the neck skin was predominantly intact, so that incision in those areas was not necessary.

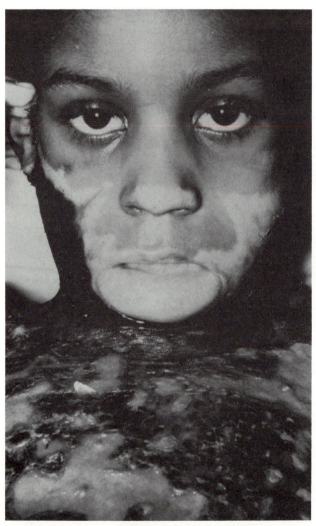

Figure 22-10

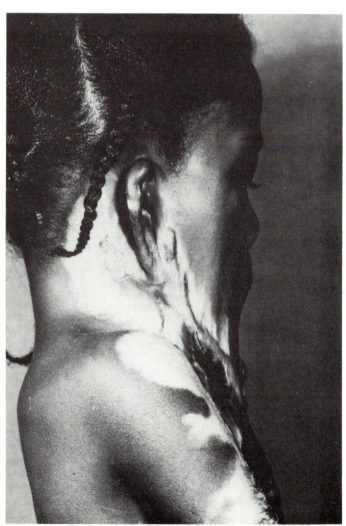

Figure 22-11

CERVICAL CONTRACTURE INVOLVING THE ENTIRE ANTERIOR SURFACE OF THE NECK

Figures 22-13, 22-14. The upper and lower incisions are indicated. No excision of intervening tissue was required since the initial injury had destroyed the skin between the mandibular margin and thorax, and these areas had become approximated during the process of healing and contracture. Dissection is performed below, through the plane established in the upper dissection, until full extension of the neck is possible. Medium-thickness skin grafts (0.014 inches) were taken from available donor sites over the upper gluteal areas, and transferred to the large cervical defect. A bulky, circumferential occlusive dressing was applied over the sutured grafts.

Figure 22-15. Fourteen days after surgery, a molded plaster splint with a thin, protective, foam rubber lining was used for support of the neck in extension, and to apply pressure to the healing grafts. The patient tolerated this type of splint well. Today, a lighter, more easily adjustable splint made of heat-labile, plastic material would be used. A continuous splinting program was carried out for a period of 11 months.

After the period of splinting, plans were outlined for revision of the vermilion-lower lip-chin facial unit, but the child's parents refused further surgery.

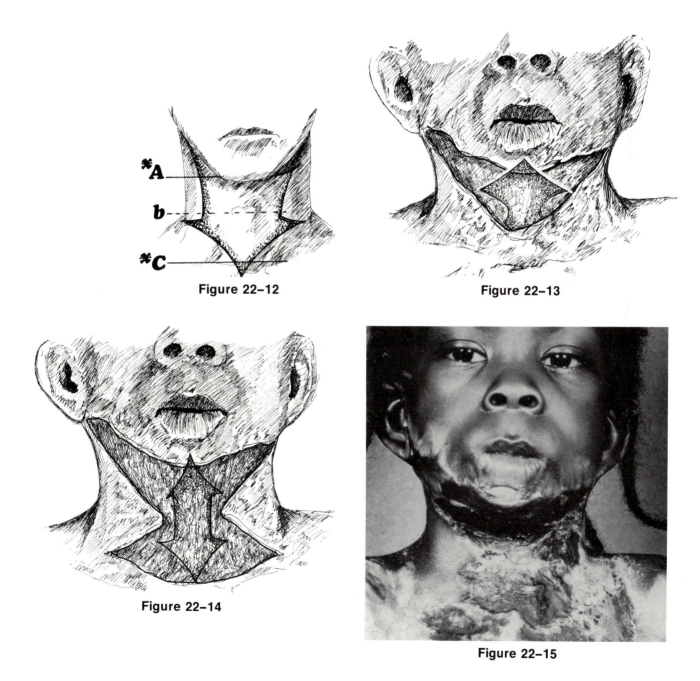

Figure 22-12

Figure 22-13

Figure 22-14

Figure 22-15

Figures 22-16, 22-17. The same patient is shown, nine years after release and resurfacing of the anterior neck. There has been excellent maintenance of the cervicomandibular angle, and reasonable positioning of the facial structures. A further offer of revision of the ectropion of the lower lip was made, but was refused by the parents and the patient.

Pitfalls and Solutions

1. In massive anterior cervical contractures, preoperative planning in consultation with the anesthesiologist is mandatory. Repeated attempts at blind and difficult endotracheal intubation, or even intubation under direct vision, may result in laryngeal trauma and laryngospasm, necessitating emergency tracheostomy.

2. The amount of hemorrhage from dissection of large cervical contractures can be extensive. Preoperative arrangements for blood replacement, particularly in the pediatric patient, should be made routinely.

3. Incisions should not encroach upon upper facial esthetic units unless excision of hypertrophic scar in these areas is absolutely necessary. Frequently it is possible to note improvement of such areas of scarring after tension from below is relieved.

4. Prolonged periods of postoperative splinting are required. Patient compliance must be encouraged often and firmly, to maximize the results in terms of range of motion of the neck and improved esthetic appearance.

CERVICAL CONTRACTURE INVOLVING THE ENTIRE ANTERIOR SURFACE OF THE NECK

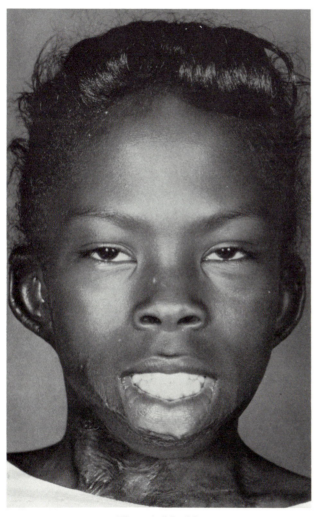

Figure 22–16

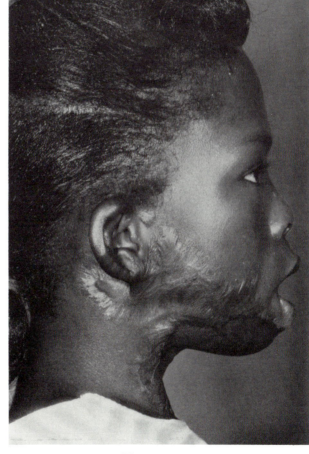

Figure 22–17

23

Cervical Contracture Below the Level of the Hyoid

The Problem

Scar contracture in the lower cervical region, below the level of the hyoid bone, often occurs in association with healed anterior thoracic burns. The submandibular area itself is occasionally uninvolved. When the upper neck and face are spared with respect to scarring, a localized release may be suitable, since the patient can cover the lower neck areas with normal clothing.

Technique

Figures 23-1, 23-2. This patient had massive body burns, with scarring almost entirely limited to below the midcervical region. The lateral cervical areas were normally pliable and uninjured. A Z-plasty repair of this localized, vertical scar was not elected because the tissue at, and below, the junction of the neck and thorax (*inset at *C*) was rigid and hypertrophic. An incision at the junction of the neck and thorax (*C) is made to preserve the relatively pliable upper cervical skin.

Figure 23-3. The dissection, which in this case was required deep to the platysma muscle, allowed upward and downward release of the anterior neck. Full extension of the neck must be gained at surgery. Meticulous hemostasis is obtained by frequent discontinuation of the dissection, and electrocoagulation of bleeding vessels.

Figure 23-4. A medium split-thickness skin graft (0.016 inches) is taken from the scalp and sutured into position. This patient had a minimal donor site area below the clavicles. Furthermore, the color and texture match of scalp grafts with cervical skin is more appropriate than that of grafts taken from other sites. The sutures of 5-0 monofilament material used to stabilize the skin graft are left uncut, so that they may be tied over an occlusive bolster for support of the wound.

CERVICAL CONTRACTURE BELOW THE LEVEL OF THE HYOID

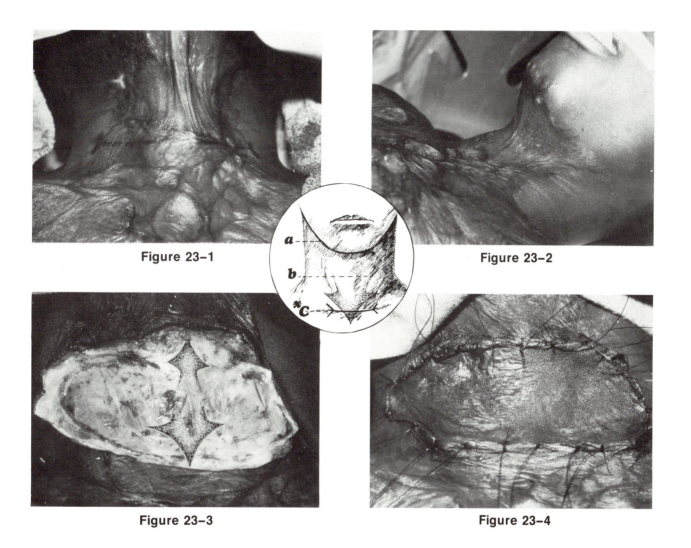

Figure 23-1

Figure 23-2

Figure 23-3

Figure 23-4

103

Figures 23-5, 23-6. The early result, with elimination of the vertical band of scar contracture that restricted neck extension, is seen. After ten days of early skin graft healing, a molded, heat-labile, plastic splint is made, lined with foam material, and applied to maintain pressure and extension of the neck. This patient would not comply with the long splinting program that is required for optimal results. The late appearance of the skin graft and surrounding tissues was not appreciably different from that seen in this photograph. However, the contour of the neck, the cervicomental angle, and the extension of the neck were adequate.

Pitfalls and Solutions

1. Incision and dissection of burn scars in the cervical region result in considerable hemorrhage. Hemostasis is mandatory prior to resurfacing with skin grafts. If hemostasis is in doubt, grafting should be delayed for 24 to 48 hours.

2. Failure to achieve an adequate long-term splinting program will lead to an unsatisfactory functional and esthetic result.

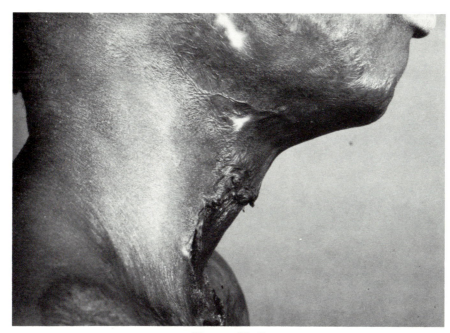
Figure 23-5

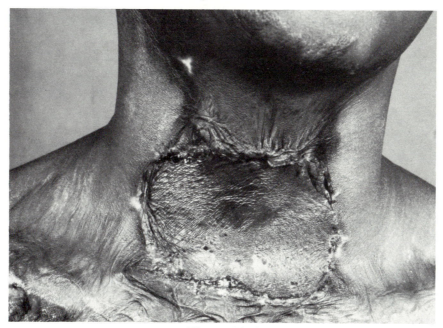
Figure 23-6

Upper Extremity

24

The Axilla

The Problem

The commonest axillary deformities following burn injuries are:
   a. Anterior only, with web formation.
   b. Anterior and posterior, with webs, the fossa or cupola being spared.
   c. Total axillary scarring or obliteration.
   d. Vertical scar extending over the deltoid, limiting abduction.
   e. Unburned, but shortened, axillary web of skin between scars of the upper arm and chest.

Technique

A Z-plasty or an advancement flap is ideal for the narrow scar contracture. However, the surrounding skin often is scarred and the injury may have extended to muscle, leaving no well vascularized skin or soft tissue available for flaps.

Figure 24-1A, B. A linear contracture that initially appeared amenable to flap reconstruction was surrounded by thick scar and healed skin grafts.

Figure 24-2. Incisions must be extended anteriorly and posteriorly until all skin tension that is preventing full abduction or extension is released. Release by incision resulted in a very large defect even before the full passive range of motion was achieved.

Figure 24-3. If the defect requires several drums of split-thickness skin graft, the suture lines should be oriented transversely to avoid another contracture.

Figure 24-4. One year postoperatively, the patient has full abduction of both arms.

Figure 24-5A, B. If only the anterior and posterior borders of the axilla are burned, and the hair-bearing cupola is spared, the surgeon must remember that the structure is dome-shaped, and contracture may occur vertically and/or horizontally. A single incision across the center is inappropriate if the cupola has been spared by the burn, because this would result in hair-bearing skin being moved onto the arm or chest. Two incisions and grafts may be most appropriate at the axilla-chest and arm-axilla junctures, relieving the contracture, but keeping the hair in the normal location.

THE AXILLA

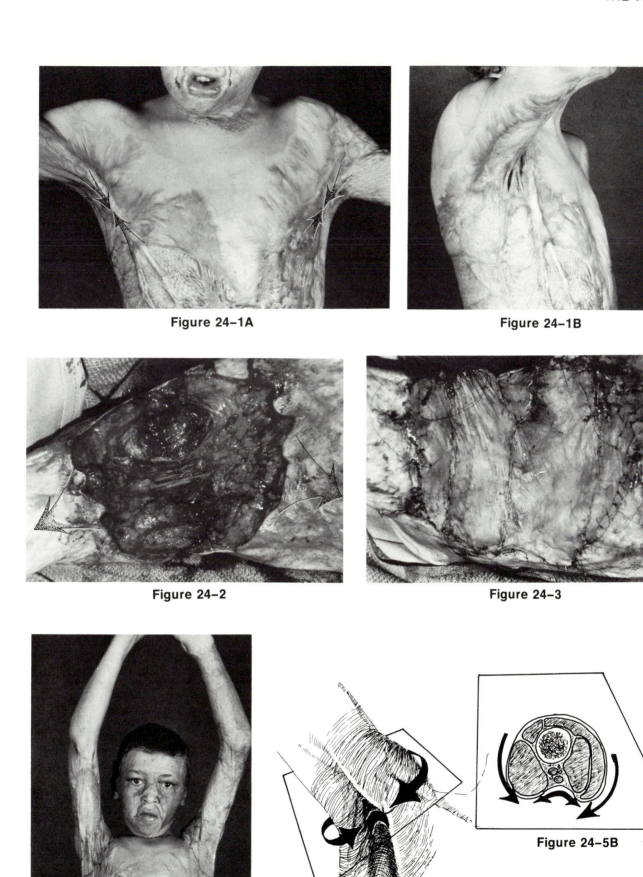

Figure 24-1A

Figure 24-1B

Figure 24-2

Figure 24-3

Figure 24-4

Figure 24-5A

Figure 24-5B

109

UPPER EXTREMITY

Figure 24–6A, B. If only the anterior axilla is contracted, the posterior, unburned tissue may be advanced as a flap into the defect after it is incised, avoiding a skin graft. Local advancement flaps, rather than incision and grafting, were chosen; this child formed keloids in previous wounds, and the possibility of keloid formation in skin graft donor sites was thus avoided. The nonhealing ulcer was outlined and excised. A broad flap based on the posterior axillary fold was outlined and raised from the underlying fascia. If the pectoralis fascia and muscle are contracted, preventing full passive or active abduction of the arm, they must be incised.

Figure 24–7. The flaps are secured in place with half-buried mattress sutures tied over cotton bolsters.

Figure 24–8. The postoperative position for splinting is always less than at the limit of passive extension of the elbow or abduction of the shoulder, so that there is no tension on the healing flap.

Figure 24–9A, B. After several weeks, full passive and active motion of the elbow and shoulder were obtained.

Pitfalls and Solutions

1. If the incisions are not extended far enough anteriorly and posteriorly, complete release of the arm and shoulder will be impossible to achieve.

2. Do not hesitate to cut contracted fascia over the pectoralis major and latissimus dorsi muscles if this is the cause of limitation of motion.

3. When the skin graft is bolstered in place, and with the patient still anesthetized, apply an abduction splint to limit postoperative motion.

4. If skin grafts have been used, the patient must wear a splint continuously for six months, and then nightly for three more months. The natural position of the arm at rest is in abduction, so that too early splint removal leads to recurrence of contracture. If reconstruction is performed using a flap, three months of continuous splinting is usually adequate.

5. Early postoperative recurrence after an adequate release usually means the splint has not been worn. The situation can be salvaged only by admitting the patient to the hospital and using serial splinting for several days. If unsuccessful, continuous traction on a radial, transosseous pin, with a yoke, pulleys, and weights, will often recover the lost range of motion. Once a recurrent axillary contracture has become fixed, only reoperation and appropriate splinting will correct it.

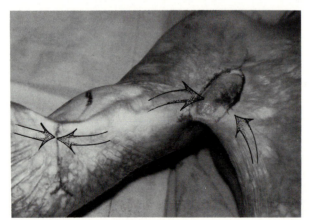

Figure 24–6A

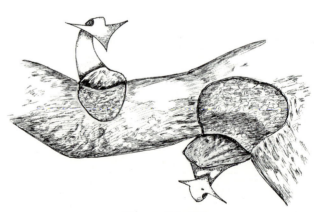

Figure 24–6B

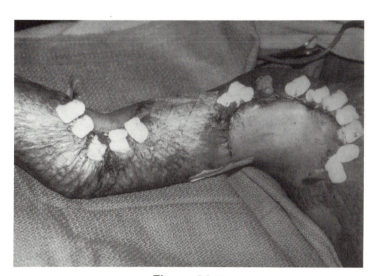

Figure 24–7

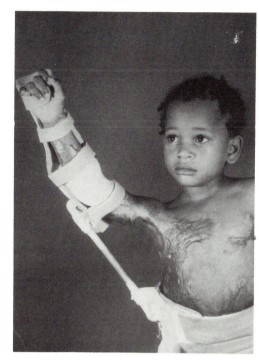

Figure 24–8

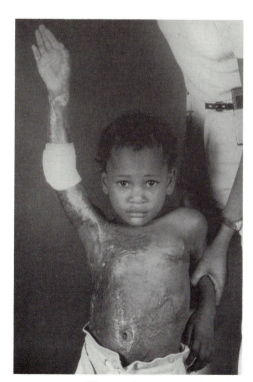

Figure 24–9A

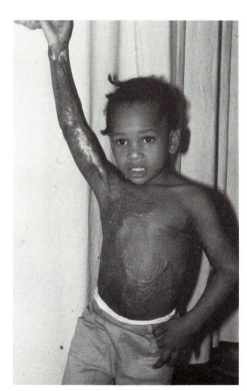

Figure 24–9B

25

Management of Elbow Contractures

The Problem

Contractures at the elbow may be corrected by:
a. Distant flaps.
b. Excision and skin graft.
c. Incision and skin graft.
d. Local advancement flaps.

Distant flaps are necessary only when the contracture is long-standing and there has been extreme shortening of the biceps tendon, median nerve, and joint capsule. In this instance, a lateral thoracicoabdominal flap may be appropriate to provide adequate tissue to cover a tenotomy, neurolysis, and capsulotomy.

Excision and skin graft is rarely indicated, because even an unsightly scar in this area can be covered by a sleeve. Only for the patient with a recurrent, nonhealing ulcer, or one whose acute injury was small and who has minimal need of skin for reconstruction, is it worthwhile to sacrifice a donor site for this purpose. Finally, when tension is released in an elbow contracture, splinting and pressure dressings usually smooth out an unsightly scar.

Incision and skin graft is most often utilized, and when combined with appropriate postoperative splinting is usually successful. The most common error is not doing a complete release. Specifically, to get full extension, one often must cut superficial veins, fascia, and even part of the biceps.

Technique

Figure 25–1A, B. This 21-year-old male, two years following injury, has a 90-degree flexion deformity.

Figure 25–2. The procedure should be done with a pneumatic tourniquet in place to improve visualization of important structures, such as the median nerve. The incision is shown with a dart at each end that converts the shape of the wound from an ellipse to a rectangle bounded with two V-shaped flaps, decreasing the chance for recontracture. The recurrent ulcer in the midline is excised.

Figure 25–3. Release is incomplete when the incision is carried through the superficial soft tissue only.

Figures 25–4, 25–5. Complete release follows incision of the contracted fascia and some biceps muscle.

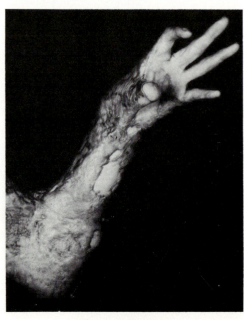

Figure 25–1A

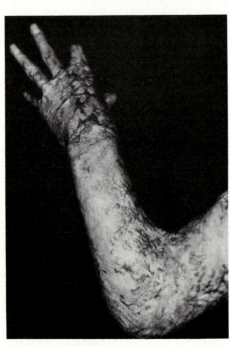

Figure 25–1B

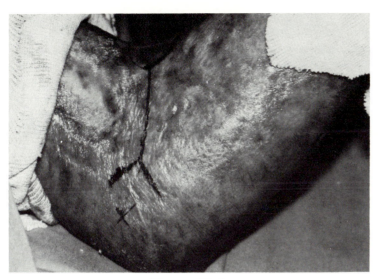

Figure 25-2

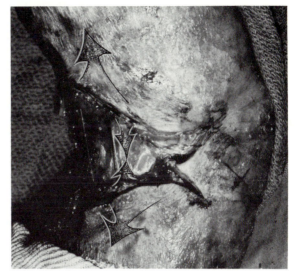

Figure 25-3

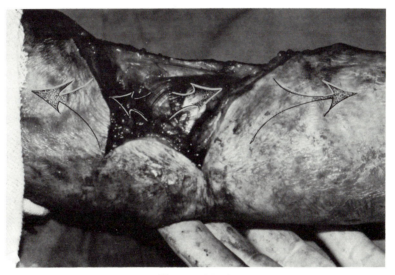

Figure 25-4

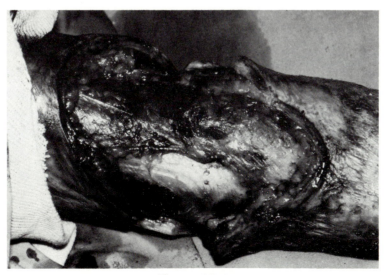

Figure 25-5

UPPER EXTREMITY

Figure 25–6. Several drums of split-thickness skin (0.018 to 0.020 inches thick) may be necessary to cover the resultant defect.

Figure 25–7. Postoperatively, the patient is able to extend his arm fully.

The use of local advancement flaps to correct a contracture is obviously very desirable because: (a) it moves normal soft tissue into the area of scar, making recurrence less likely; and (b) it avoids a skin graft donor site. This technique is applicable only if the scar band is narrow and if ample unburned local tissue is available.

Figure 25–8. The mid- and lateral antecubital fossae are completely unburned, and the hypertrophic scar band is discrete and narrow, making an advancement flap feasible.

Figure 25–9. The narrow band to be incised has been marked, and the broad advancement flap outlined. It is imperative that the tip be rounded and the base of the flap be as broad as possible to preserve its blood supply. Once the scar band is incised, the flap is elevated from the muscular fascia, because bleeding will be minimal and the maximal thickness of soft tissue can be moved into the defect. Care should be taken to protect the venous drainage of the flap. Only veins that restrict flap mobility should be cut. It is neither necessary nor advisable to undermine the base of the flap initially.

Figure 25–10. Using a skin hook, one should check the tension of the advancement flap periodically to see when enough elevation and advancement has been achieved, and to stop the dissection at that point.

Subcutaneous closure is performed with buried, inverted, absorbable sutures. Running, subcuticular monofilament or half-buried mattress sutures are used on the skin. If, when straightening the elbow, the flap seems under tension in its new position, the surgeon must undermine the base further to gain length, and place the elbow temporarily in slight flexion temporarily until healing has occurred. The elbow is mobilized progressively into extension several weeks after surgery. In the rare case in which the extent of contracture has been underestimated, a supplementary skin graft may be used.

Figure 25–11. It is advisable to overcorrect the defect by advancing the flap as far beyond the midline of the contracture as possible.

Pitfalls and Solutions

1. Avoid injury to the median nerve when making the transverse incision at the elbow. The nerve may be more superficial in the contracted tissue than is immediately appreciated.

2. Flaps under tension necrose. When flaps that are too small are stretched to cover a larger defect, ischemia and tissue death result.

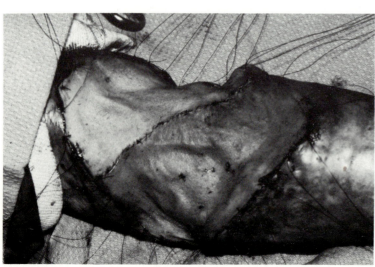

Figure 25–6

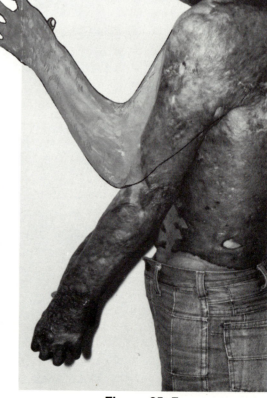

Figure 25–7

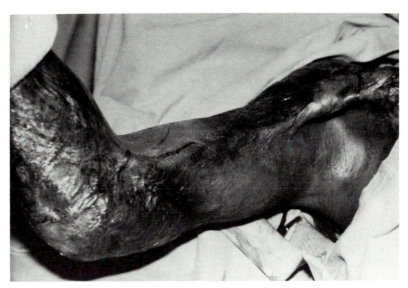

Figure 25–8

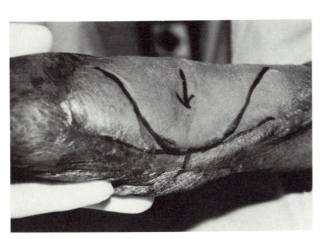

Figure 25–9

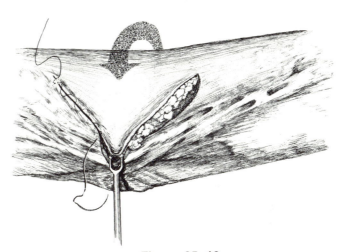

Figure 25–10

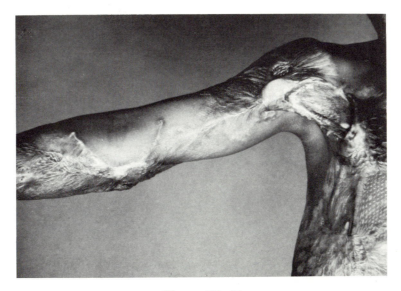

Figure 25–11

26

Peripheral Nerve Loss Secondary to Electrical Injury

The Problem

In high-amperage electrical injury, peripheral nerves are often destroyed. Current follows the path of least resistance, and nerve has the least resistance of all tissue.

When confronted with a patient desiring reconstruction, the surgeon has four alternatives:
  a. No operative treatment because of other medical priorities.
  b. Nerve reconstruction.
  c. Tendon transfers or selective arthrodeses.
  d. Amputation.

Occasionally the severity of the systemic injury is such that peripheral nerve reconstruction has a very low priority and may be delayed indefinitely.

Figure 26-1. For instance, this exit wound over the medial condyle destroyed the ulnar nerve, but no reconstruction was done because the patient also had destruction of the posterior scalp, skull, and both legs, necessitating bilateral above-knee amputations. Several episodes of pulmonary embolism made it necessary to achieve ambulation as soon as possible.

Figure 26-2. The patient needed both arms to move on canes, and nerve reconstruction would have confined him to a chair or bed. Most important, he was not hindered clinically by the loss of sensation or power in the distribution of the ulnar nerve. Thus, no attempt at nerve reconstruction was made.

For the patient who *is* a candidate, nerve reconstruction may include:
  a. End-to-end suture.
  b. Nerve graft.
  c. Neurolysis.
  d. Neurovascular island transfer.

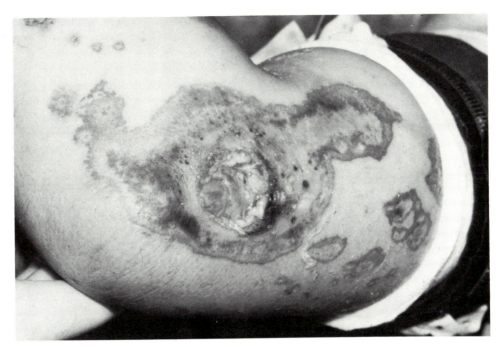

Figure 26-1

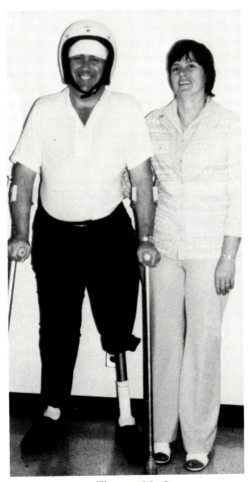

Figure 26-2

The Problem

End-to-end repair following electrical injury is rarely possible because long segments of nerve are usually damaged, and it requires great tension to bring them together once the damaged portion is resected. Nerve grafting is an option in these cases and is indicated when:

a. There is a long enough history of clinical loss to rule out neurapraxia.

b. There is confirmation of nerve deficit by nerve conduction and/or electromyographic studies.

Technique

Figure 26-3. This scarred wrist resulted from an electrical injury that destroyed the sensory branch of the radial nerve. The patient was an electrician, and the anesthesia hindered him on his job. He desired reconstruction, and the exploratory skin incision was curvilinear so that no longitudinal scar would overlie the nerve repair.

Figure 26-4. The sensory nerve above the tape had areas of replacement by longitudinally oriented scar. With magnification, resection of the damaged nerve was performed proximally and distally to where normal fascicles were apparent. The length of the deficit was too great for end-to-end repair, and a graft was indicated.

Figure 26-5. Technique of sural nerve graft removal:

The sterile field should include both legs, in case the donor graft from one leg is too small or is damaged during removal. The longitudinal incision at the lateral ankle is made carefully in soft tissue between the Achilles tendon and lateral malleolus (marked with an "X" on this cadaver leg). The nerve is identified and a tape is placed beneath it. The nerve is superficial, and no structures of importance are in danger of being cut inadvertently. Multiple transverse or longitudinal incisions are made proximally until the desired length of nerve is dissected free. The transverse lines indicate the medial course of the nerve. Tension should not be placed on the nerve, or it will be damaged. Although some surgeons use a stripper for removing the sural nerve, there is a real danger of cutting the nerve prematurely, making it too short, or damaging it by traction.

Figure 26-6. The wrist is placed in neutral position and slight radial deviation, and the sural nerve graft inserted. (By properly positioning the hand first, the graft will not be made too long or too short.) Depending on the diameter of the recipient nerve, one, two, or three cables are used. Quadrant sutures of 9-0 monofilament material are inserted through the epineurium. The repair is done without tension. Immobilization in a hand dressing and splint is accomplished with the wrist in the neutral position.

Pitfalls and Solutions

Too short or too long a graft will not help the patient at all. It is imperative to place the hand in a neutral position, and tailor the graft to the gap.

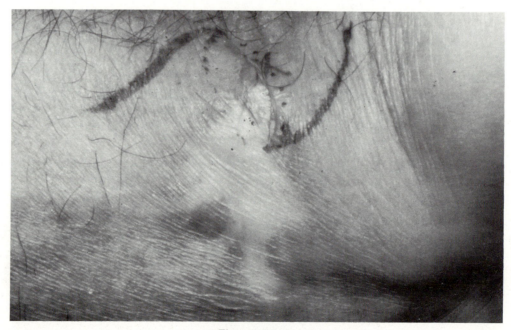

Figure 26-3

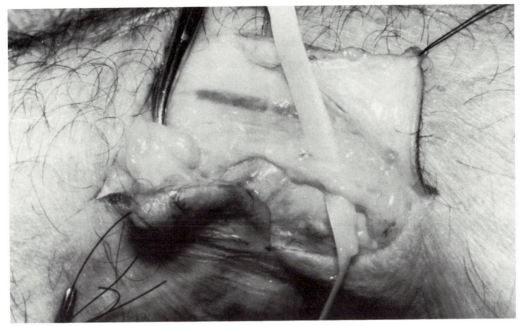

Figure 26-4

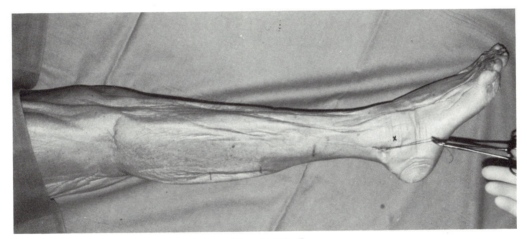

Figure 26-5

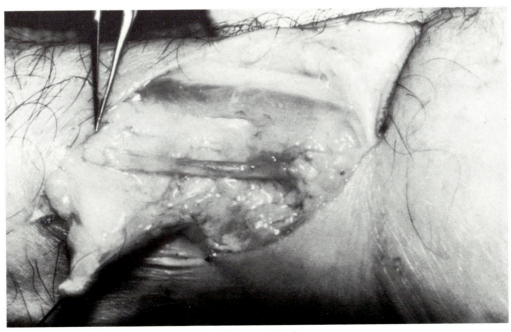

Figure 26-6

UPPER EXTREMITY

The Problem

Occasionally, exploration of the nerve reveals a situation that can best be salvaged by neurolysis.

Figure 26–7. This patient's right arm was destroyed by high-voltage electricity. An exit wound injury of the left wrist resulted in decreased sensation and paresthesias along the course of the median and ulnar nerves.

Technique

Because a skin graft has been applied to the left wrist wound, the incision was made through the scar, and dissection above the paratenon maintained maximal thickness of the flaps.

Figure 26–8. Before the neurolysis is begun, a tape is placed under the nerve to facilitate its manipulation in the wound.

Figure 26–9. Using magnification, the epineurium is incised. The surgeon and assistant each grasp an edge and dissect it from the nerve, gently teasing fascicles from the scar. With the assistant also holding the epineurium, the chance of cutting a fascicle as the nerve is freed posteriorly is decreased. Although there is evidence that excessive dissection increases the chance of more scar formation, fascicular neurolysis must be complete.

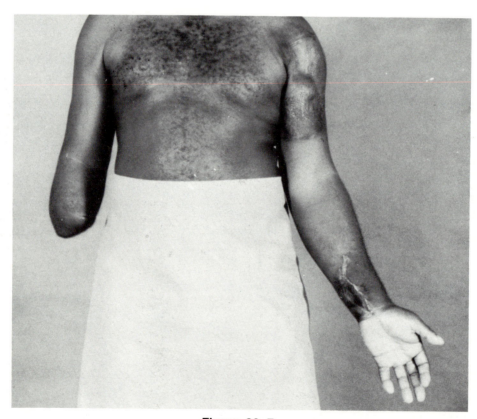

Figure 26–7

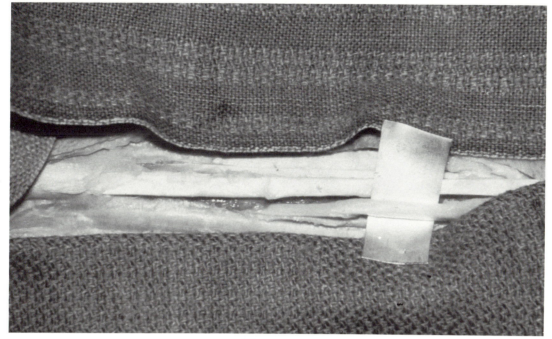

Figure 26-8

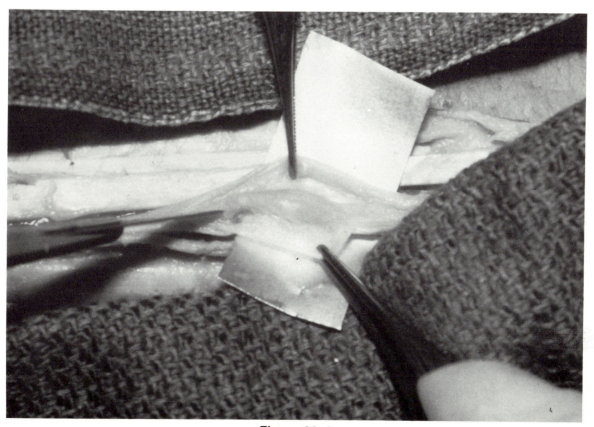

Figure 26-9

UPPER EXTREMITY

Pitfalls and Solutions

1. The neurolysis must extend proximally and distally to normal tissue, or the constriction will not be alleviated.

2. Once external neurolysis has been done, individual fascicles should be examined under magnification to be certain they have been released. If not, fascicular neurolysis is mandatory.

The Problem

Figures 26-10, 26-11. Occasionally, electrical neurovascular injury impairs the ability to pinch. In this case, the radial digital neurovascular bundle of the index finger was destroyed, and the proximal interphalangeal joint opened. Other systemic injuries obviated the chance for early flap coverage. The patient refused amputation of the finger. Therefore, treatment included debridement, rongeuring of the bone to encourage formation of granulation tissue, and then skin grafting for temporary wound coverage.

Figure 26-12. The patient is now a candidate for proximal interphalangeal joint fusion and neurovascular island transfer from the ring finger that was uninvolved.

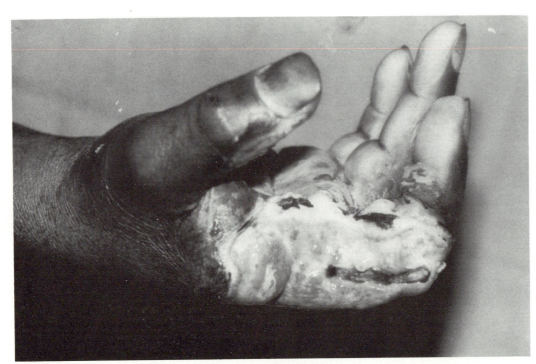

Figure 26-10

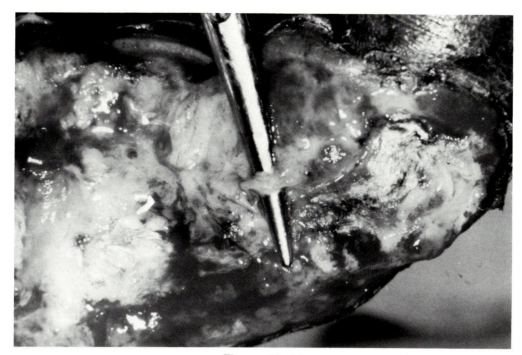

Figure 26-11

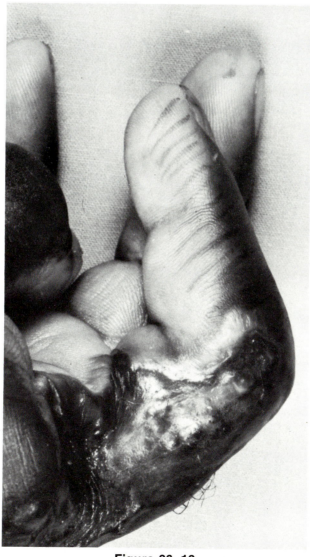

Figure 26-12

Technique

Figure 26-13. The technique of neurovascular island transfer is illustrated in another patient with a high-tension injury of the thumb that destroyed the ulnar neurovascular bundle.

Figure 26-14. Using Brilliant Green solution, a flap is outlined on the ulnar side of the long finger. The recipient site may be prepared by dermabrasion or excision with a scalpel.

Figure 26-15. The pedicle was dissected. As dissection proceeds into the palm, one must be careful to retain the proper digital artery and vein and not stretch them, or irreversible spasm may result.

Figure 26-16. To get adequate length, the surgeon ligates and cuts the proper digital artery and vein to the radial side of the ring finger at its origin from the common digital vessels. The common digital nerve was split and teased apart proximally to allow transfer without tension.

Figure 26-17. The flap is passed across the palm beneath the palmar fascia. This can be done by tunneling, taking care not to kink the vessels and nerve, or under direct vision, by making an incision parallel to the distal palmar crease.

Figure 26-18. With the thumb defect now covered, the donor site is closed with a split-thickness skin graft.

Pitfalls and Solutions

1. All dissection must be done under magnification to minimize trauma to the pedicle.
2. Stretching of the bundle must be avoided, or postoperative paresthesia and hyperesthesia will ensue.

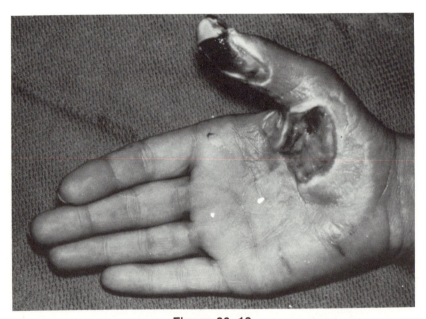

Figure 26-13

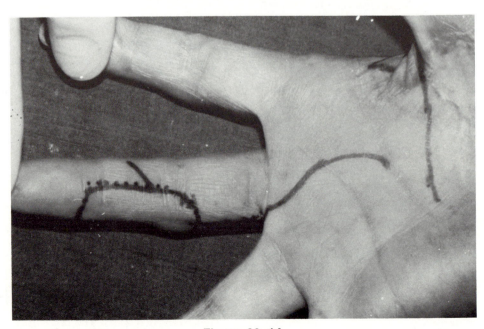

Figure 26-14

PERIPHERAL NERVE LOSS SECONDARY TO ELECTRICAL INJURY

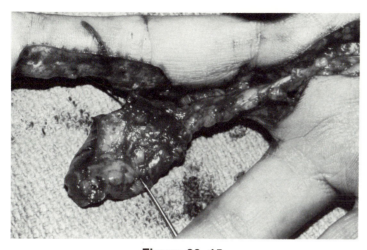

Figure 26–15

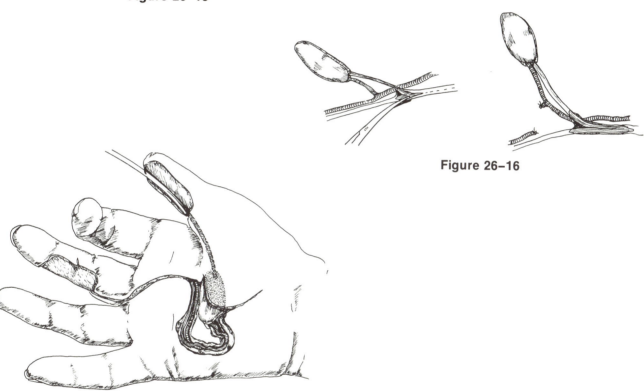

Figure 26–16

Figure 26–17

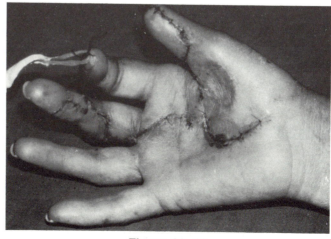

Figure 26–18

27

Heterotopic Ossification: Radioulnar Synostosis

The Problem

The etiology of heterotopic ossification between bones and across joints is unclear. Patients' serum calcium level is normal. Possible contributory causes that have been implicated include long confinement in bed, full-thickness burn, and inadequate physical therapy. A common site of involvement is the upper extremity, especially in the elbow region. Patients' presenting complaints are limitation of motion or peripheral sensory deficits.

Technique

Figure 27–1. The patient's right arm is fixed midway between supination and pronation. There is no limitation of elbow flexion or extension.

Figure 27–2. Significant ossification connecting the proximal radius and ulna distal to the elbow joint is seen.

Figure 27–3A, B. With the elbow flexed, the drawing indicates that the area of ossification was not in proximity to the ulnar nerve in this patient. Because of the location of heterotopic ossification, it is not necessary to operate over the joint, and a simple, linear incision in the posterior midline of the arm will suffice. A pneumatic tourniquet is used during the dissection.

Figure 27–4. Retraction of soft tissue reveals the pathological ossification.

Figure 27–5. The abnormal bone can be excised with an osteotome or rongeur. Note that the ulnar nerve is identified and gently retracted with a rubber tape. Even though the radiograph strongly suggested that there was no ossification in the region of the ulnar nerve, anatomical variance is possible, and preliminary identification of the nerve allows the surgeon to proceed further without fear of injuring it.

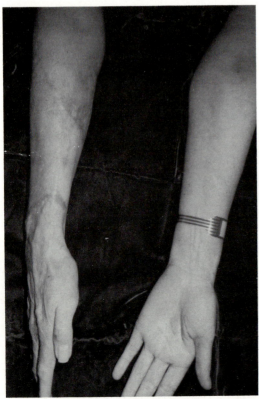

Figure 27–1

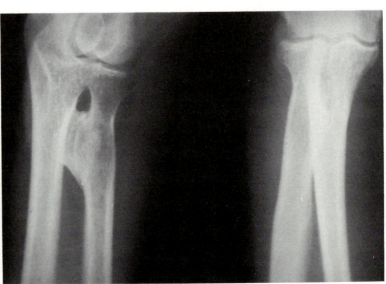

Figure 27–2

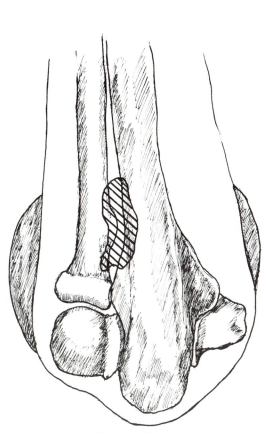

Figure 27-3A

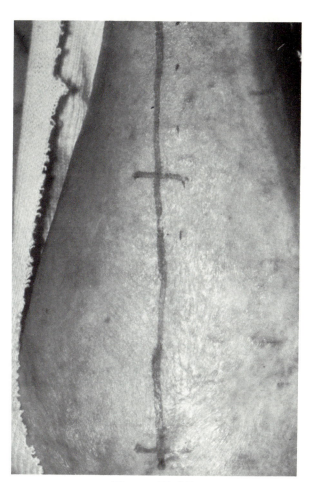

Figure 27-3B

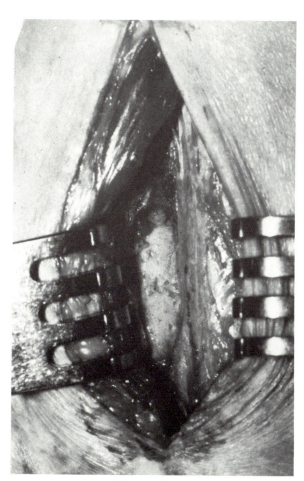

Figure 27-4

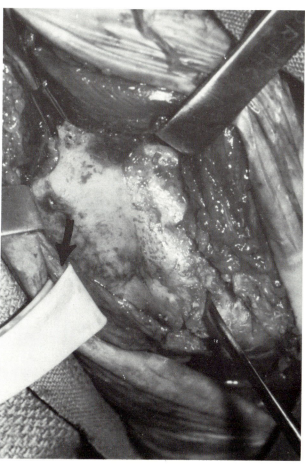

Figure 27-5

UPPER EXTREMITY

Figure 27-6. **A**, Resection of the ossification must be as complete as possible, or limitation of motion will persist. Any remaining pathological bone should be rasped free of sharp spicules.

B, The operative wound is shown, revealing the absence of abnormal bone after excision. No fascia or synthetic material is interposed between the radius and ulna, as there is no proof that this retards recurrence.

Figure 27-7A, B. Radiographs made several months postoperatively reveal no recurrent ossification in this patient, and the range of motion is now complete, with normal pronation.

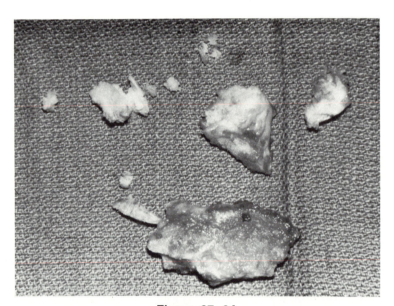

Figure 27-6A

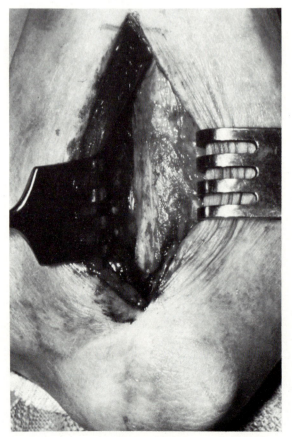

Figure 27-6B

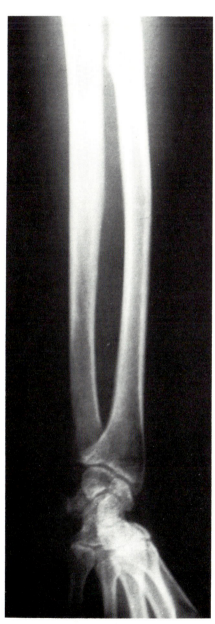

Figure 27–7A

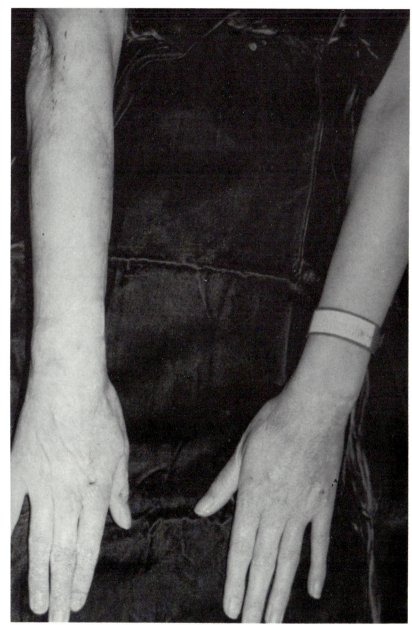

Figure 27–7B

UPPER EXTREMITY

Figure 27-8. Frequently the abnormal ossification will extend posteriorly and surround the ulnar nerve. In this patient the presenting complaints were limitation of elbow motion, with sensory and motor dysfunction due to ulnar nerve compression. There is great risk of injuring the nerve at surgery because its position in the ossification is unpredictable.

Figure 27-9. The incision must be made to permit identification of the ulnar nerve proximal and distal to the pathologic condition. In the upper half of the arm the ulnar nerve lies medial to the brachial artery, but at midarm it goes through the intermuscular septum to pass in front of the medial head of the triceps. It descends posterior to the medial epicondyle of the humerus, and enters the forearm between the humeral and ulnar heads of the flexor carpi ulnaris. Usually no motor branches lie above the elbow, except an occasional one to the flexor carpi ulnaris. The nerve descends in the forearm beneath the flexor carpi ulnaris, and lies over the flexor digitorum profundus. Branches of the nerve near the elbow that must be protected include: (a) articular branches, at the level of the elbow; and (b) muscular branches to the flexor digitorum profundus that lie near the level of the medial epicondyle.

Figure 27-10. Fine rubber tapes are placed around the ulnar nerve so that it is always visible in the operative field. Using a rongeur, bits of abnormal bone are excised along the course of the nerve. It is unwise to use an osteotome until the nerve is completely exposed and retracted. Pursuing the ossification may lead into the elbow joint, but the procedure should not be terminated until the ulnar nerve is freed and a satisfactory range of elbow motion is obtained.

Postoperatively, splinting should position the elbow in mild flexion. The forearm is held in supination or pronation (reversing the preoperative deformity).

Range of motion exercises may begin one week following surgery, and should be supervised by a therapist to ensure patient compliance. If the extremity has been disabled for a long time, it may be difficult to achieve early mobilization because of muscle fibrosis and joint capsule contracture.

Pitfalls and Solutions

1. If there is any question of ulnar nerve entrapment, it should be identified proximal and distal to the area of pathology, and dissected free of the ossification.

2. Even after meticulous resection of heterotopic ossification and diligent postoperative mobilization, occasional recurrence is noted. All patients must be advised of this possibility preoperatively.

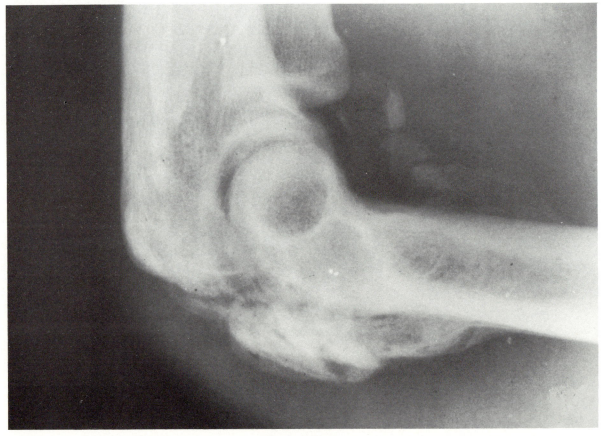

Figure 27-8

HETEROTOPIC OSSIFICATION: RADIOULNAR SYNOSTOSIS

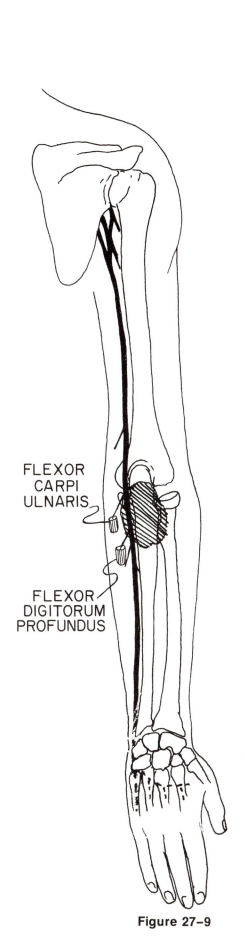

Figure 27-9

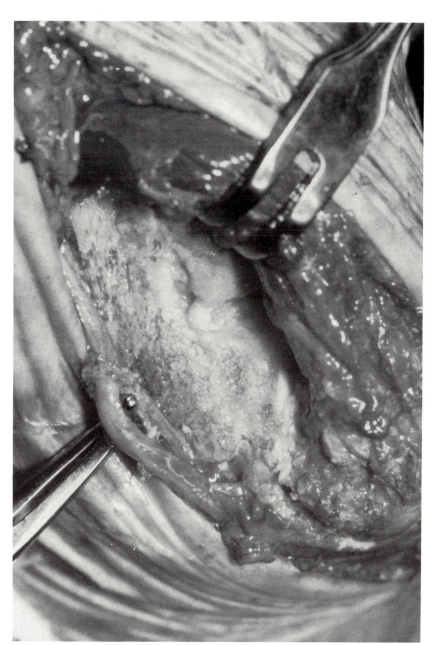

Figure 27-10

28
Dorsal and Volar Wrist Contractures: Abduction of the Thumb

The Problem

Most authors have emphasized the need for appropriate splinting after the release of contractures of the fingers or palm, or following excision of dorsal scarring of the hand. The wrist is rarely mentioned, however, as it is assumed by some that the action of the powerful wrist flexors and extensors will always prevent contracture formation. Unfortunately, no matter how elegant the surgery, the hand must be splinted in an overcorrected position for nine to 12 months following release of scar contracture and skin grafting, or recurrence is predictable.

Technique

Figure 28–1. This severe dorsal contracture, holding all fingers and the wrist in hyperextension, resulted from inadequate skin graft coverage.

Figure 28–2. A large defect results when the scar is excised. The metacarpophalangeal joints are pinned in 60 degrees of flexion.

Figure 28–3. Postoperative splinting maintains the wrist in neutral position during the day when the patient is using the hand, and in flexion at night. Dynamic finger traction, using an outrigger with finger cuffs, holds the metacarpophalangeal joints in flexion.

Figure 28–4. Failure to wear the splint has resulted in contracture of the wound. Note the patient's inability to achieve full finger flexion when the wrist is flexed slightly, owing to tightening and inadequate length of the dorsal skin cover.

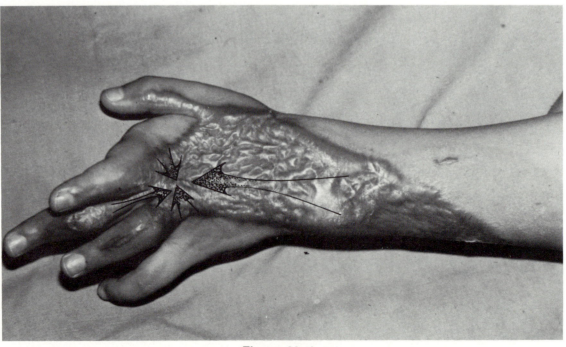

Figure 28–1

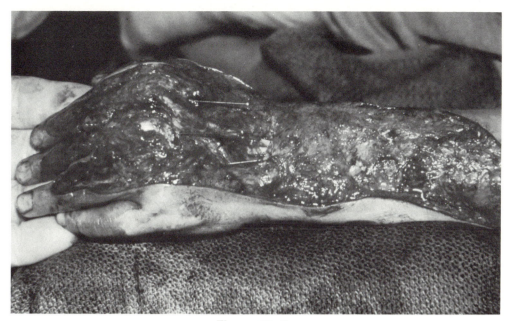

Figure 28-2

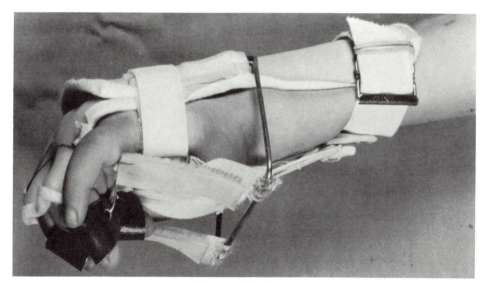

Figure 28-3

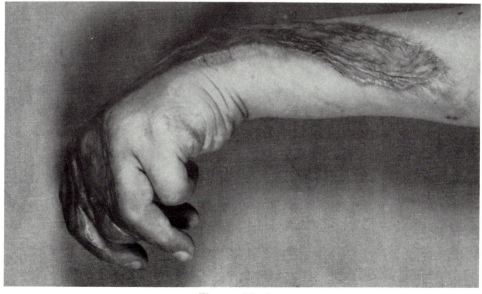

Figure 28-4

UPPER EXTREMITY

The Problem

Dorsal contractures over the first digital web and radial surface of the distal wrist have produced an abduction deformity of the thumb. The thumb is rendered useless for pinch and grasp.

Figure 28-5. Scar contracture at the base of the thumb has pulled it into abduction and extended the first metacarpal. Scar is also present over the dorsum of the thumb-index web space.

Technique

Figure 28-6. Transverse incision of the scar is performed down to the level of the intact paratenon of the extensor pollicis longus and brevis and the abductor pollicis longus muscles. Usually the paratenon will be intact, and must be maintained to provide an adequate recipient site for split-thickness skin grafts. A similar incision is made in the thumb-index web scar, which also divides any tight fascia overlying the adductor pollicis muscle. Care is taken not to injure any branches of the dorsal radial nerve. Further, soft tissue dissection in the thumb-index web must be cautious, avoiding injury to the radial digital neurovascular bundle to the index finger, and to the neurovascular structures supplying the thumb. The thumb is released in all planes until there is full range of motion of the metacarpal base. Split-thickness skin grafts (0.016 inches) are applied, and sutured with monofilament material. Frequently a transosseous Kirschner wire is passed axially through the thumb, fixing it in extension and mild abduction as if it were an extension of the radius. The hand is placed in occlusive dressing and maintained in elevation.

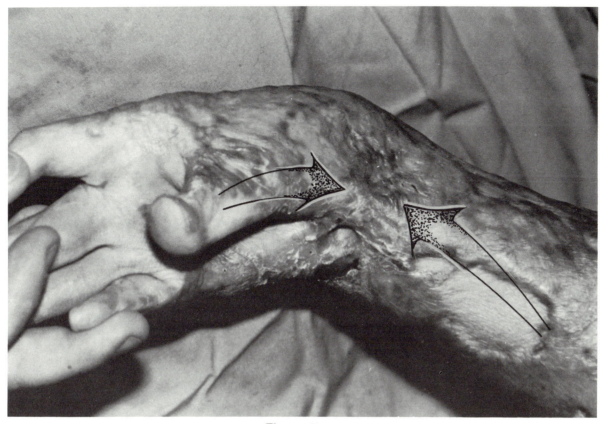

Figure 28-5

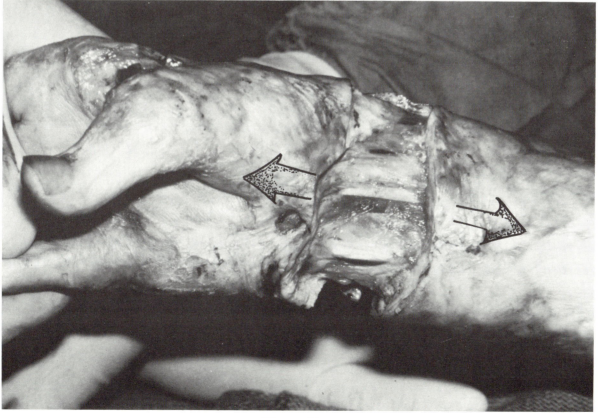

Figure 28-6

Figure 28–7. Ten to 12 days postoperatively the management of the hand includes removal of the transosseous wire, a fitted pressure glove, and a molded splint to hold the thumb in mild abduction. The wrist is moved into more extension gradually, to avoid injury to the median nerve by traction.

Figures 28–8, 28–9. Several weeks later the wrist is in extension, the thumb-index space is adequate for grasp and pinch, and correction of the abduction contracture involving the thumb metacarpal base is achieved.

Pitfalls and Solutions

1. If splinting is not begun in the operating room and maintained postoperatively, contracture of the grafted wound can occur and will not be overcome by wrist flexors or extensors.

2. Do not cut the paratenon and attempt to graft denuded tendon, or skin graft failure will result.

3. Injury to sensory branches of the radial nerve in the dorsal tissues of the first web area will result if indiscriminate dissection is done.

4. Dissection deep in the soft tissue of the first web must be done with care, as the neurovascular structures to the thumb and radial side of the index digit course directly through this area on its palmar surface.

5. If the metacarpophalangeal joint of the thumb is extended or hyperextended after release of the metacarpal base, capsular contracture has ensued and must be treated by capsulotomy. The capsule of the metacarpophalangeal joint must be incised, and the joint immobilized with a Kirschner wire in neutral extension or 15 degrees of flexion.

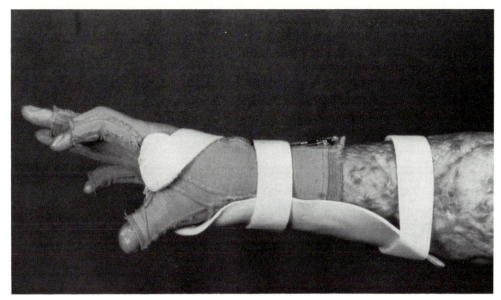

Figure 28-7

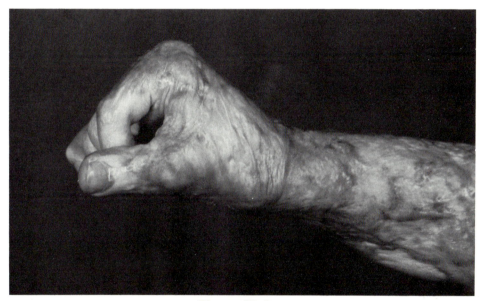

Figure 28-8

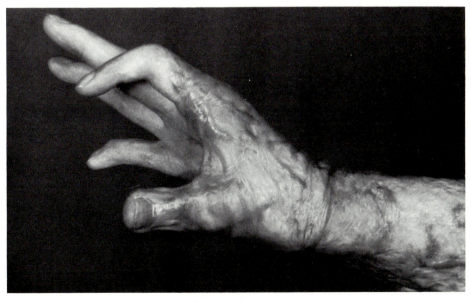

Figure 28-9

29

The Metacarpal Hand: An Opposable Cleft

The Problem

In the multiply traumatized patient, a hand without fingers can still perform valuable "assistive" functions in support of the good hand. Depending on the patient's age, occupation, associated injuries, and expectations, either multiple operative procedures or none at all may be performed. Although a prosthetic device supplies pinch and would be quite suitable for the anesthetic hand, the presence of excellent sensibility encourages an attempt to achieve pinch surgically.

Technique

Figure 29–1. A hand is illustrated in which all fingers are absent at the metacarpophalangeal joint level, but palmar breadth is adequate. Sensibility was excellent, but no grasp was possible. Radiographs revealed that only a small portion of the index metacarpal remained (from an earlier debridement).

Figure 29–2. A linear S-shaped incision is made to open the first web space fully.

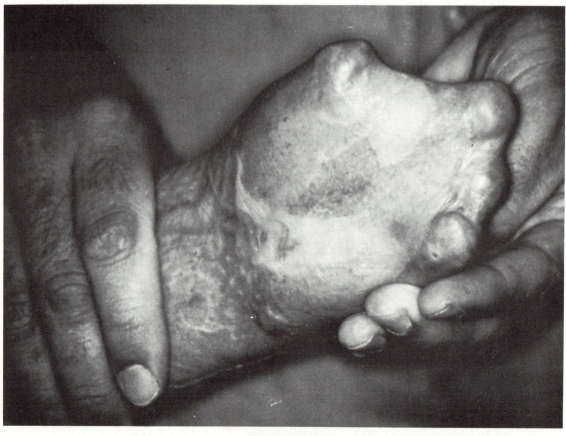

Figure 29–1

Figure 29–3. To achieve complete release, a tight, scarred adductor pollicis muscle must be incised subperiosteally at its insertion on the first metacarpal, taking care to leave some fibers intact to preserve its important function.

Figure 29–4. Any contracted fascia overlying the muscle is incised and released. The long metacarpal is excised at the level of the neck to further widen the cleft. Excision is performed subperiosteally to retain adductor function. No attempt is made to excise redundant soft tissue, as it will remodel and provide excellent padding during grasp. A split-thickness skin graft (0.018 to 0.020 inches) is used to cover the wounds, and is held in place with a bolstered, tie-over dressing to prevent hematoma formation.

Figure 29–5. Postoperatively, the patient demonstrates a satisfactory breadth of grasp for small and moderately large objects.

Pitfalls and Solutions

1. Release must be complete in the operating room. Postoperative therapy will maintain, but not necessarily increase, the surgical gains.

2. The skin graft must be thick to give durability during pinch and grasp. Thin grafts here may lead to a hypersensitive scarred wound.

3. The open wound is often deep and convoluted. The dressing over the skin graft must conform to the new web space, so that the skin graft will be held in full approximation to the wound; otherwise, hematoma and further scarring will result.

4. The adductor pollicis muscle is released by subperiosteal incision over the third metacarpal. If the muscle is stripped from the bone extraperiosteally, or dissected grossly, a functionless, fibrotic muscle results, and pinch and grasp are compromised.

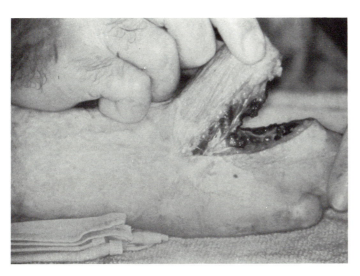

Figure 29–2

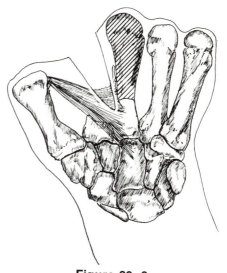

Figure 29–3

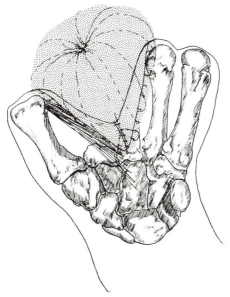

Figure 29–4

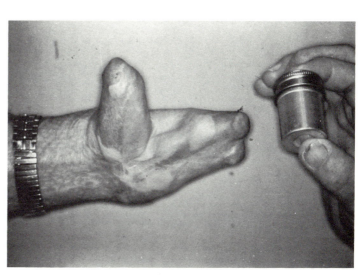

Figure 29–5

30

The Accessory Hand: Selective Amputation

The Problem

Although amputation of an injured digit is usually the least desirable alternative for the hand surgeon, problems of the upper extremity must always be considered in the context of the rest of the patient's burns. Since there often are other reconstructive procedures with higher priority, and time constraints with regard to returning the patient to work or school, amputation should always be considered when:

a. There is severe skin, soft tissue, joint, and neurovascular injury.

b. The rest of the hand functions adequately, but a digit is useless.

Technique

Figure 30–1. A severely dislocated proximal interphalangeal joint of the grafted small finger secondary to scar contracture is illustrated. The neurovascular bundles had been cut inadvertently during a previous attempt at contracture release, and there were flexor tendon adhesions. The rest of the hand healed from a deep, second-degree burn and functioned well, and the other hand was normal.

Figure 30–2. For this viable, but useless, finger, an amputation was performed at the metacarpophalangeal joint because the patient wished to return to work as soon as possible, and the chances for successful reconstruction were very questionable. A dorsal flap was used with a volar suture line. Usually it is desirable to place the suture line dorsally, away from the grasping surface, but this volar tissue consisted of unstable scar.

Figure 30–3. If the remainder of the hand is severely compromised, elective amputation is rarely considered. An amputated small finger, with volar finger flexion contractures, and hyperextension of the proximal interphalangeal joint of the long finger due to a boutonnière deformity, is illustrated. A rotational flexion deformity of the ring finger holds it in the palm, preventing the patient from grasping objects. The extensor tendon has been destroyed. In this case, the ring finger should not be amputated because it provides potentially valuable breadth to the palm.

Figures 30–4, 30–5. The incision and grafting of the volar contractures of the ring finger and proximal interphalangeal joint fusion in mild flexion have yielded an open palm, with adequate breadth that allows for grasping and holding objects. Further reconstruction is indicated for the other deformities.

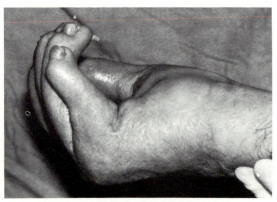

Figure 30–1

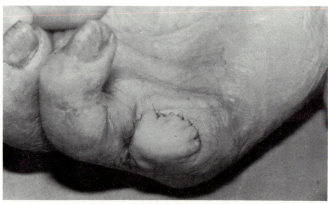

Figure 30–2

THE ACCESSORY HAND: SELECTIVE AMPUTATION

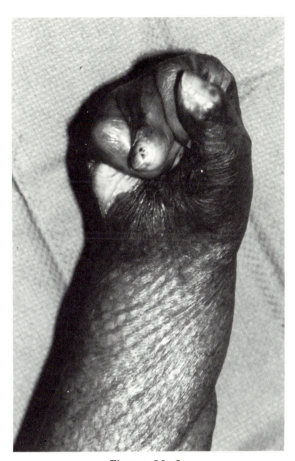

Figure 30-3

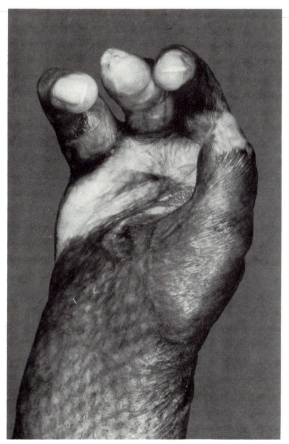

Figure 30-4

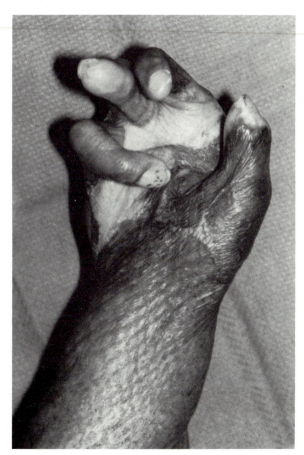

Figure 30-5

UPPER EXTREMITY

Figure 30–6. In another case a high-voltage electrical injury has destroyed volar skin and soft tissue of the thumb distal to the metacarpophalangeal joint, as well as bone, flexor tendons, and neurovascular bundles. Only part of the dorsal skin bridge has survived.

Figure 30–7. The small finger had the same tissue loss demarcated, and both were amputated in addition to the nonviable long finger. The index finger, however, was salvageable since, although volar skin and soft tissue were destroyed, tendon and neurovascular bundles were only injured.

Figure 30–8. Because of the other amputations, it is very important to salvage this finger. The hand is held against the chest to test for a comfortable position. After a pattern is cut to the size of the defect, the random flap is drawn with a 1:1 or 2:1 ratio. Chest skin is thin, and a flap that has little fat, and is not bulky, can be raised. Both the thumb stump and the index digit were covered with the flap in the hope of providing good soft tissue for pain-free pinch. The stump of the small finger was skin-grafted. The pedicle was separated two weeks later and, employing the "crane principle," a thin layer of soft tissue was left that was skin-grafted.

Figures 30–9, 30–10. Satisfactory coverage and function were achieved.

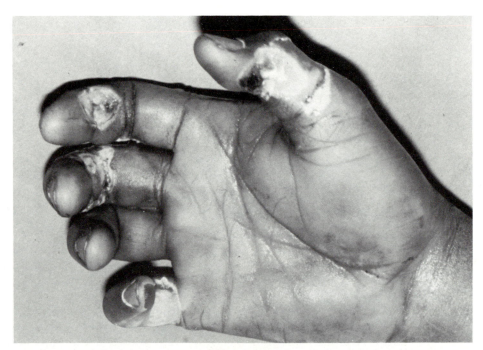

Figure 30–6

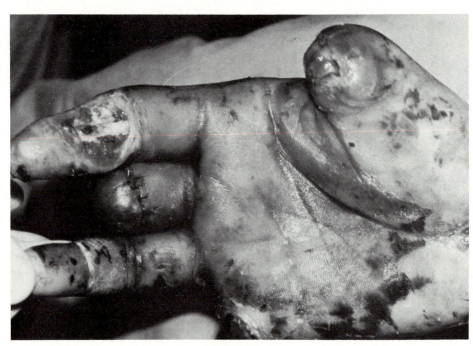

Figure 30–7

THE ACCESSORY HAND: SELECTIVE AMPUTATION

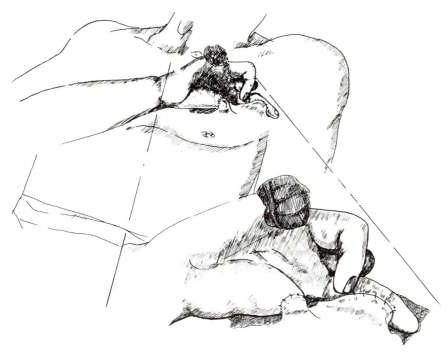

Figure 30-8

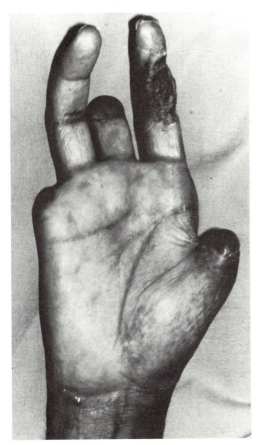

Figure 30-9

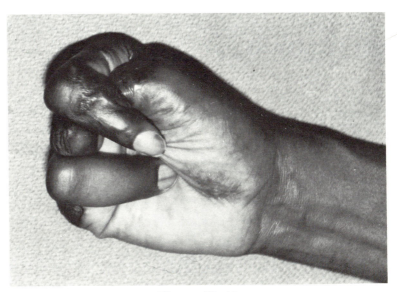

Figure 30-10

31

Excision and Grafting of the Dorsum of the Hand

The Problem

Excision and grafting of the dorsum of the hand is indicated for the problems illustrated in Figures 31–1 and 31–2.

Figure 31–1. Healed, deep, second-degree burns with unstable skin that ulcerates frequently.

Figure 31–2. Healed, deep, second-degree or grafted third-degree injury that has resulted in very thick, hypertrophic scar that limits the range of motion. In addition to healed volar burns, this patient had Dupuytren's contracture involving the small digit.

EXCISION AND GRAFTING OF THE DORSUM OF THE HAND

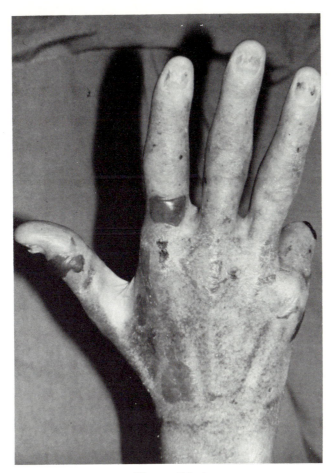

Figure 31-1

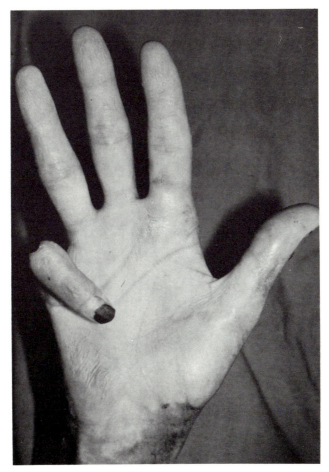

Figure 31-2

Technique

Figures 31–3, 31–4. Incisions on the digits should be marked to the extent of unstable skin, even if out to the base of the nail on the distal phalanx. Linear incisions are extended onto the midlateral plane and made V-shaped on the interdigital webs, to prevent postoperative dorsal hooding.

Figure 31–5. Excision is begun proximally, sparing the paratenon and dorsal veins. If one follows the remaining veins distally, they indicate the proper plane of dissection. The surgeon must be cautious in dissecting the interdigital webs, because injudicious probing with scalpel or scissors invariably injures too many veins and lymphatics. Difficult bleeding will result when the tourniquet is released, and may lead to obstructive venous stasis and edema of the digits.

When the excision is finished, hemostasis is achieved. The bleeding is usually brisk and the surgeon must have patience, applying whatever techniques work best for him to obtain a dry wound (pressure dressing, epinephrine-soaked sponges, electrocautery). It is helpful to apply a pressure dressing while the arm is elevated for ten minutes.

Figure 31–6. A Kirschner wire should be inserted longitudinally through the metacarpophalangeal joints after placing each one in approximately 80 degrees of flexion. It may be possible to hold the fingers in the flexed position in a soft dressing without wire fixation, but more reliable fixation is achieved *with* it. With the wrist and metacarpophalangeal joints placed in flexion before applying the skin graft, the wound surface area will be stretched maximally so that an adequate amount of skin graft is applied.

Figures 31–7, 31–8. Note in these photographs, taken 14 days postoperatively, that the skin grafts are applied so that the suture lines are all transverse or oblique, to avoid longitudinal scar contractures.. The grafts are tailored so that the suture lines do not lie over joints. In this manner, if any graft failure results, tendon and/or joint spaces are not exposed. (Local excision of the palmar fibromatosis present in this patient, and release of the flexion contracture, necessitated a volar skin graft.) Skin graft junctures are secured with adhesive strips and/or a continuous 6-0 synthetic, absorbable suture.

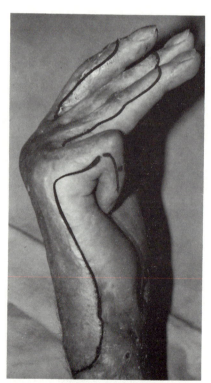

Figure 31-3

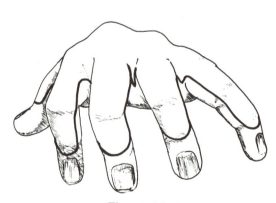

Figure 31-4

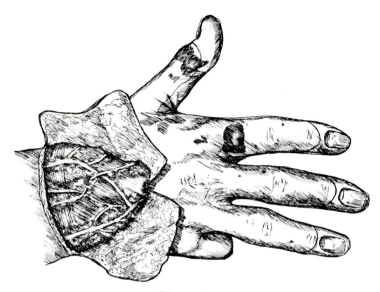

Figure 31-5

Figure 31-6

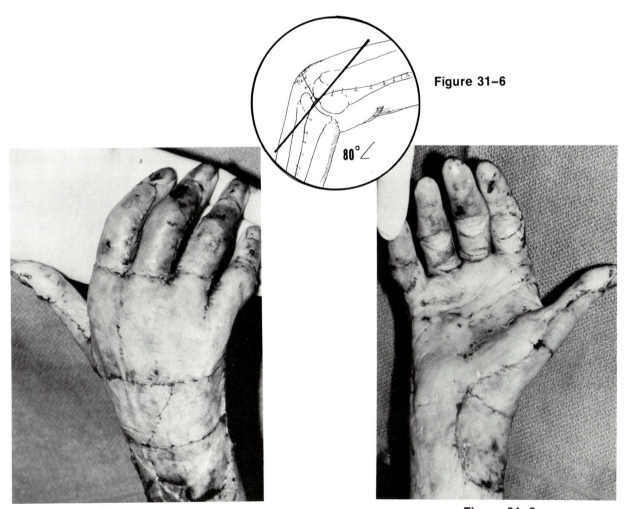

Figure 31-7

Figure 31-8

UPPER EXTREMITY

Figures 31–9, 31–10. The skin grafts should be moderately thick (0.021 inches), to decrease the amount of wound contraction that may occur. Six months postoperatively there are no dorsal or volar ulcerations, indicating that the skin is indeed serviceable under stress, and apparently durable.

Figures 31–11, 31–12, 31–13. For the dorsal wound that oozes regardless of attempts at hemostasis, some surgeons choose to apply a dressing for 24 hours and then return to the operating room again for skin grafting. Another alternative is to mesh the skin grafts 1.5 to 1. The graft is thus "pie-crusted," and not stretched significantly. Collection of blood or serum beneath the graft is uncommon under these circumstances. Hypertrophic scarring is no more of a possibility with meshed skin graft than with intact sheet grafts, as long as the mesh is applied without expansion. In these postoperative views of maturing, meshed skin graft, there is a rich network of dorsal veins, and lack of edema. There is no hypertrophic scar, full extension and flexion is possible, and the skin is supple and yielding.

Pitfalls and Solutions

1. Incisions should be begun in normal tissue, to identify the proper plane of dissection. Indiscriminate dissection and disruption of dorsal veins and lymphatics will result in an edematous hand.

2. Incisions in the fingers should lie midlaterally whenever possible, and not volarly, or they may lead to flexion contracture.

3. Always deflate the tourniquet and patiently achieve hemostasis before grafting. Hematoma may compromise the entire operative result.

4. Thick skin grafts must be employed to achieve better functional results. Meshed skin grafts are useful in the difficult wound in which hemostasis is in doubt even after diligent efforts.

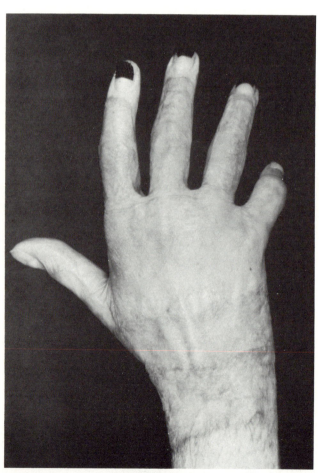

Figure 31–9

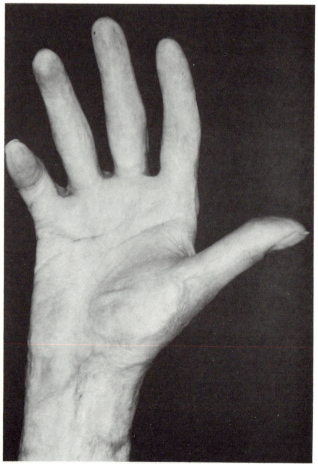

Figure 31–10

EXCISION AND GRAFTING OF THE DORSUM OF THE HAND

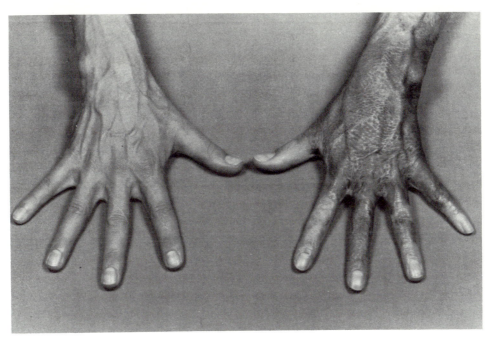

Figure 31-11

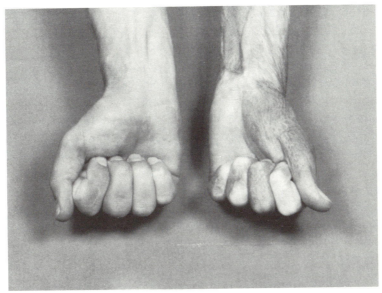

Figure 31-12

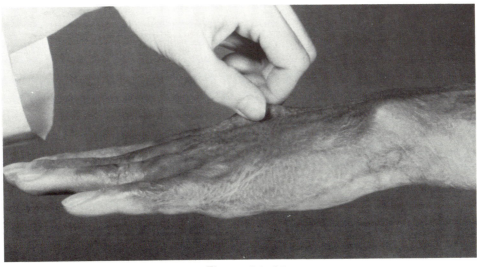

Figure 31-13

32

Palm and Finger Contractures

The Problem

Morbidity from a deep burn involving the dorsum and palm is much greater than with the isolated dorsal burn. Most surgeons do not primarily excise the burned palm because:

a. There is no edematous, bloodless plane, as may be found on the dorsum.

b. The excellent sensibility and durability of the palmar skin are unique, and worth preserving if at all possible.

Figure 32–1. One sequela of a palmar burn may be a severe contracture, as illustrated, with all fingers drawn into marked and fixed flexion.

Figure 32–2. The effect of contraction not only restricts flexion and extension, but also narrows the breadth of the palm.

Although excision and grafting is possible, it is extremely bloody, and graft healing is as difficult as when one attempts excision of palmar fibromatosis (grafting frequently must be delayed for 24 to 48 hours to insure hemostasis). Incision and thick, split-thickness skin graft coverage of the resulting defect is often preferable, and the released skin usually remodels with time, becoming more durable and slowly acquiring better sensibility.

PALM AND FINGER CONTRACTURES

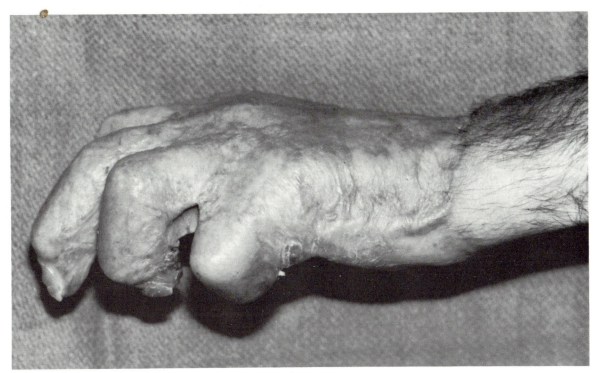

Figure 32-1

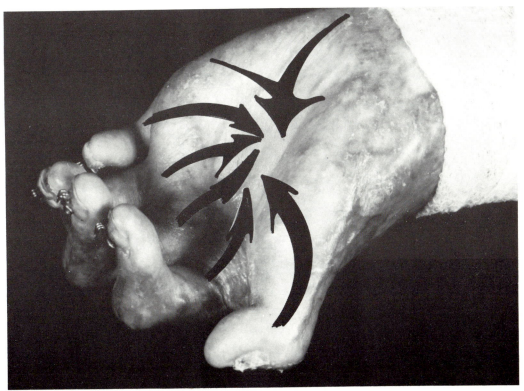

Figure 32-2

151

UPPER EXTREMITY

Technique

Figure 32-3. Before the fingers are released, the midlateral axis of the digits should be marked as a guide to the location of the neurovascular bundles. The prospective incision is transverse, ending in Y-shaped darts.

Figures 32-4, 32-5. With the pneumatic tourniquet elevated, the neurovascular bundles are identified, and the flexor tendons are isolated with a tape. The nerve and artery may look like scar bands, and may be inadvertently cut. All dissection should be performed in a longitudinal direction to avoid cutting or avulsing the vessels and nerves.

Figure 32-6. The open wounds result from incision and release, not excision, indicating the large area of deficient soft tissue. Neurovascular bundles have shortened, and sudden stretching with the tourniquet inflated could produce vascular spasm and necrosis of the fingers. If the contractures are severe, the tourniquet should be released before any attempt is made to straighten the fingers. Extreme, sudden stretching of nerves results in paresthesias and possible permanent fibrosis. Thus, when the tourniquet is released and hemostasis is achieved, the fingers are slowly extended and observed for circulatory impairment. If blanching occurs, attempts at passive extension are discontinued, and the fingers slowly flexed to that point at which good color returns. In this situation, any remaining lack of extension will have to be corrected by gradual postoperative splinting.

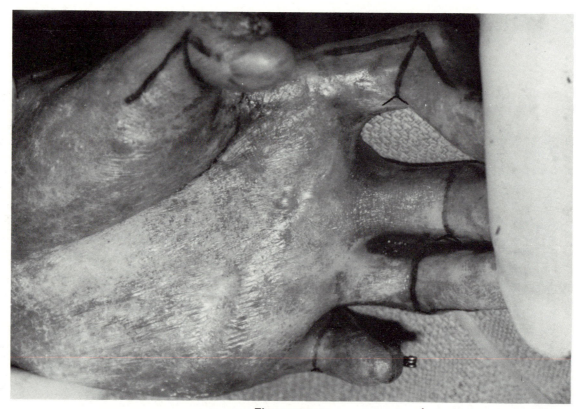

Figure 32-3

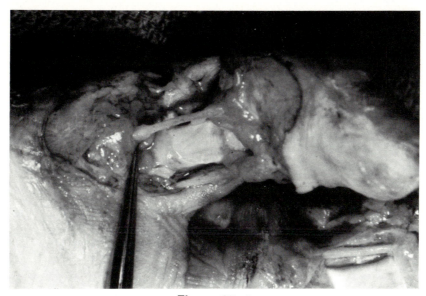

Figure 32-4

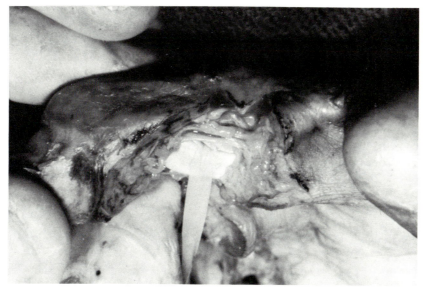

Figure 32-5

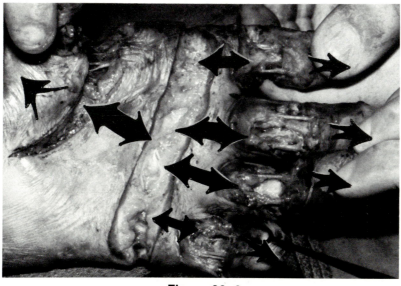

Figure 32-6

Figure 32–7. Kirschner wires placed longitudinally across the proximal interphalangeal joints maintain the correction, and should not be removed until 14 to 21 days postoperatively. The split-thickness skin grafts are held in place with a minimal number of sutures, because the reactive hyperemia after tourniquet deflation results in annoying bleeding caused by each pass of the suture needle. The dressing is not tied over a bolster, but a bulky, soft dressing is applied carefully and the extremity is splinted, with the wrist and all finger joints in extension for three weeks. When the Kirschner wires are removed, a dynamic splint should be worn during the day, keeping the palm and fingers in extension, and allowing active flexion. A simple, static extension splint can be used at night.

Figures 32–8, 32–9. One year later, finger extension and palmar breadth are improved, resulting in a more functional "assist"-type hand.

Pitfalls and Solutions

1. The neurovascular bundles must be identified positively when incising the fingers, as scar contracture may have pulled them into an abnormal position.

2. Do not extend severely contracted fingers while the tourniquet is inflated, or spasm of the shortened vessels and traction injury to nerves may result.

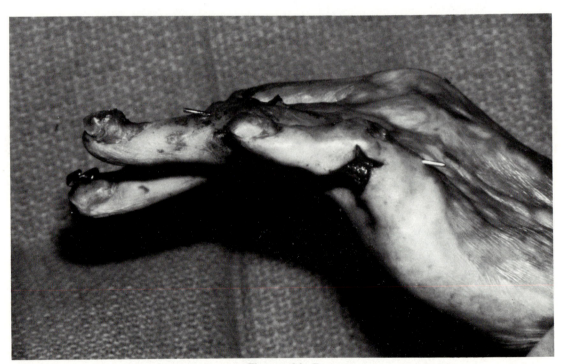

Figure 32–7

PALM AND FINGER CONTRACTURES

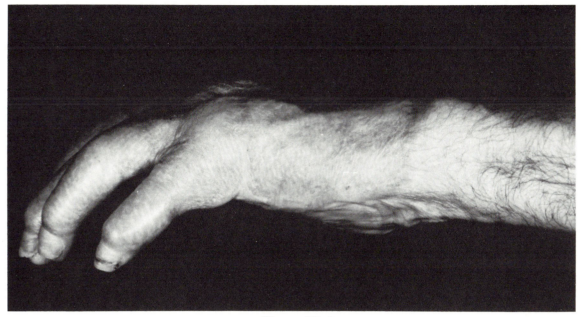

Figure 32–8

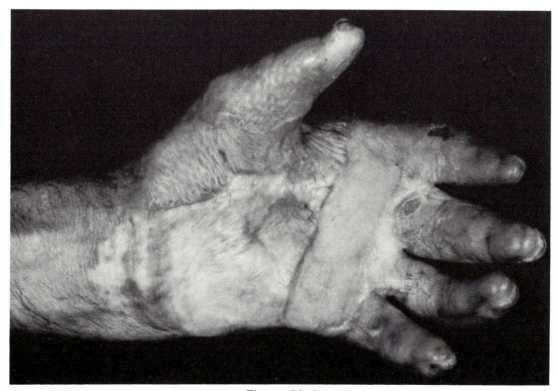

Figure 32–9

33

Metacarpophalangeal Capsulotomy and Proximal Interphalangeal Arthrodesis

The Problem

Deep burn injury to the thin dorsal skin and soft tissues over the small joints of the hand, and inadequate splinting and exercise, can lead to deformity.

Figure 33–1. There is hyperextension of the metacarpophalangeal joints and flexion of the proximal interphalangeal joints, usually with hyperextension of the distal interphalangeal joints, or boutonnière deformity. Frequently this deformity can be prevented by early, continuous splinting, with the metacarpophalangeal joint in flexion and the proximal interphalangeal joint in a neutral position. Significant pressure must be avoided in these injured areas, however, and occasionally splinting alone is inadequate to prevent deformity. If the injury is deep or if the positioning of the fingers is long-standing, the supporting structures of the metacarpophalangeal and interphalangeal joints become shortened and scarred, so that normal function is lost.

Technique

Metacarpophalangeal joint capsulectomy is required in order to reposition the hyperextended joints.

Figure 33–2A. By using individual longitudinal incisions, the injury to venous and lymphatic structures that might arise with single transverse incisions is avoided. With transverse incisions, reapproximation is often impossible, requiring the addition of skin grafts to this area when metacarpophalangeal joints are placed in flexion.

B, A longitudinal incision is made through the skin and scar contracture, and a similar one is continued through the central extensor mechanism, exposing the joint capsule. The extensor is retracted and shortened, and the contracted dorsal capsule is excised in a transverse axis, exposing the joint space and allowing passive flexion. In the hyperextension deformity the lateral bands lie above the axis of rotation of the metacarpophalangeal joint, and are contracted in a foreshortened position.

METACARPOPHALANGEAL CAPSULOTOMY

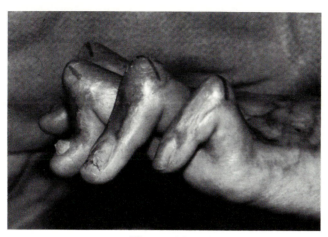

Figure 33-1

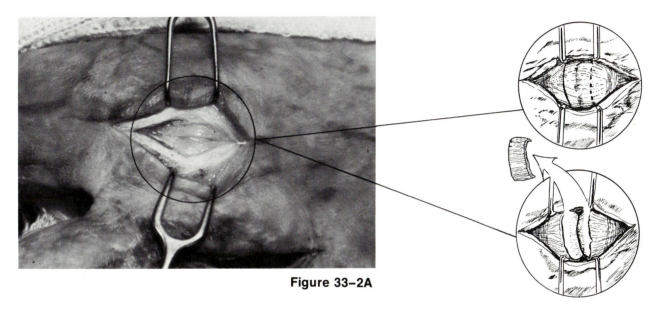

Figure 33-2A

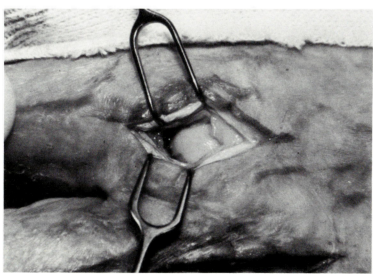

Figure 33-2B

157

Figure 33–3. The contracted collateral ligaments further impede flexion, and by using the scalpel against the metacarpal head the superior portion of the ligament is cut enough to allow passive flexion. Not all of the substance of the collateral ligaments should be divided on either side of the digit, or lateral instability will result.

Figure 33–4A, B. The volar plate adhesions are released, as described by Curtis, using a small, periosteal elevator. The volar plate is dissected proximally in order to free it from its contracted foreshortened position. The hyperextended phalanx is reduced, brought into 60 to 80 degrees of flexion, and fixed with an axial, transmetacarpophalangeal Kirschner wire. The extensor hood is repaired with several interrupted, inverted 5-0 synthetic monofilament sutures. The procedure is repeated with any other involved metacarpophalangeal joints.

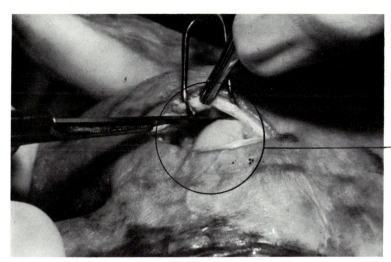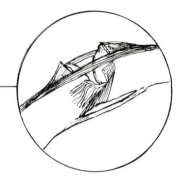

Figure 33-3

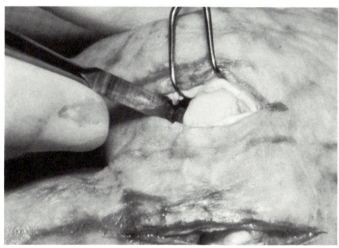

Figure 33-4A

Figure 33-4B

The Problem

Simple capsulotomy and release of the proximal interphalangeal joint flexion contractures by recession of the volar plate, division or lengthening of flexor tendons, or revision of collateral ligaments are rarely possible in the postburn injury. The injury is usually deep enough to destroy the skin and secondarily involve the central extensor mechanism. As a result, the middle phalanx becomes flexed, with hyperextension of the distal interphalangeal joint: the boutonnière deformity. Skin cover is often inadequate for ligamentous reconstruction and central extensor tendon restoration.

Proximal interphalangeal joint arthrodesis is the most effective and useful procedure to restore pinch and grasp functions.

Figure 33–5. A transverse incision is made across the proximal interphalangeal joint.

Figure 33–6A, B. The collapsed joint space and luxated middle phalanx, with absence of central extensor tendon at the proximal interphalangeal joint, are noted. Resection of the proximal head of the middle phalanx and distal portion of the proximal phalanx are done using a mechanical osteotome or narrow saw blade. The angles of the distal and proximal osteotomies are planned to accomplish two goals: (a) to allow the finger to assume a position of pulp-to-pulp pinch with the patient's opposed thumb; and (b) to achieve the greatest possible cross-sectional area of bone-to-bone apposition for successful arthrodesis.

Figure 33–7A, B. The proximal interphalangeal joint is passively positioned at a more functional angle (30 degrees of flexion) fixed with Kirschner wires.

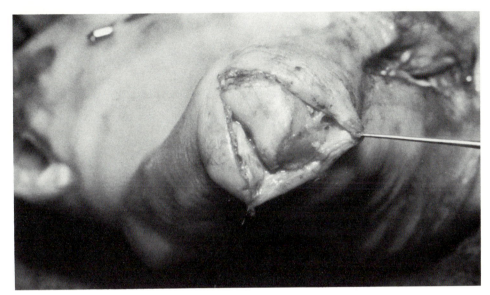

Figure 33-5

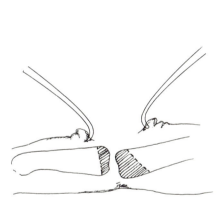

Figure 33-6A

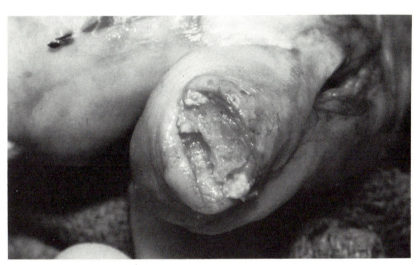

Figure 33-6B

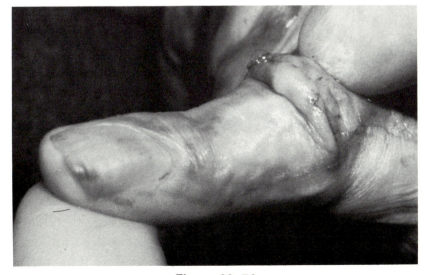

Figure 33-7A

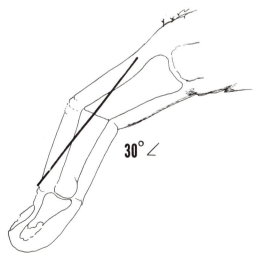

Figure 33-7B

Figure 33–8. At the completion of the procedure, the proximal interphalangeal and metacarpophalangeal joints are placed in a functional position.

Figure 33–9A, B. The patient now has a useful "assist"-type hand. The fingers no longer prevent the thumb from sweeping across the palm. They are in position for useful pinch. The distal interphalangeal joint extension deformities were not corrected at this operation.

Pitfalls and Solutions

1. Avoid complete incision of collateral ligaments, which leads to lateral instability of the digits.

2. Failure to maintain metacarpophalangeal flexion will lead to recurrence of hyperextension. This must be maintained by Kirschner wire fixation, rather than by dressings and splints alone.

3. Excellent bony contact in proximal interphalangeal arthrodesis is mandatory. Careful planning of the angles of osteotomy is required to achieve pulp-to-pulp pinch and the greatest cross-sectional area of bony apposition.

4. In patients with these types of deformities, osteoporosis and disuse atrophy of the bones is common. Following proximal interphalangeal arthrodesis, internal fixation and splinting is required for eight to 12 weeks before adequate healing occurs.

5. Edema must be avoided, since it will impede motion of the joints. Reduction of edema can be achieved by the use of intermittent occlusive dressings, pneumatic pressure devices, elevation, gradual increase in range of motion, and exercise of all unoperated joints.

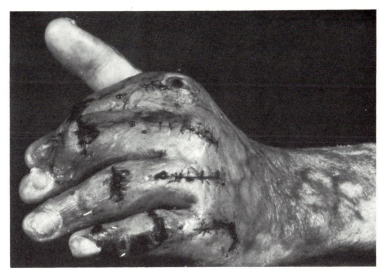
Figure 33-8

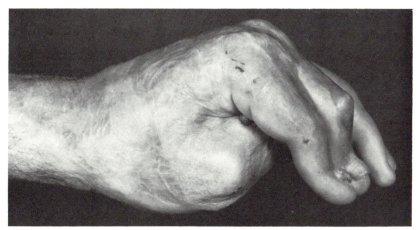
Figure 33-9A

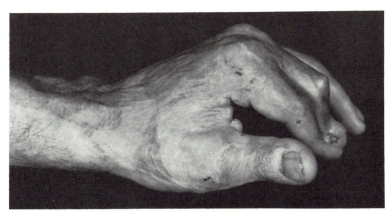
Figure 33-9B

34

Boutonnière Deformity

The Problem

The early case of boutonnière deformity is a candidate for splinting as the initial treatment (which may indeed be definitive).

Figure 34–1. All these splints attempt to diminish proximal interphalangeal joint hyperflexion and achieve some distal interphalangeal joint flexion, and are worn continuously for eight weeks. The dorsal skin of some fingers, however, will not tolerate any pressure and blistering. Frank ulceration may force abandonment of this treatment plan, making the patient a candidate for surgery.

Patients who have had boutonnière deformity for a long time, with marked dislocation of painful joints, will not respond adequately to splinting. These proximal interphalangeal joints are best treated by arthrodesis, especially when there is an associated metacarpophalangeal joint hyperextension deformity (which is treated with capsulectomy). Only a few cases of boutonnière deformity in the healed hand are amenable to definitive extensor tendon reconstruction: for example, the finger with good skin coverage and minimal joint pathology. Although many techniques have been published, Elliot's is the one that has been consistently successful in our experience.

Technique

Figure 34–2. A finger with good skin graft coverage, in a teenage patient who did not improve with splinting, is illustrated.

Figure 34–3. The pathological anatomy consists of a disrupted central slip that has migrated proximally. The lateral bands have slipped below the axis of rotation of the joint, causing proximal interphalangeal joint hyperflexion and distal interphalangeal joint extension.

Figure 34–4. A large, attenuated scar bridges the central slip, which has retracted proximally.

Figure 34–5. A small, distal cuff of scar is retained on the middle phalanx. The rest of the scar is excised proximally until normal central tendon is encountered.

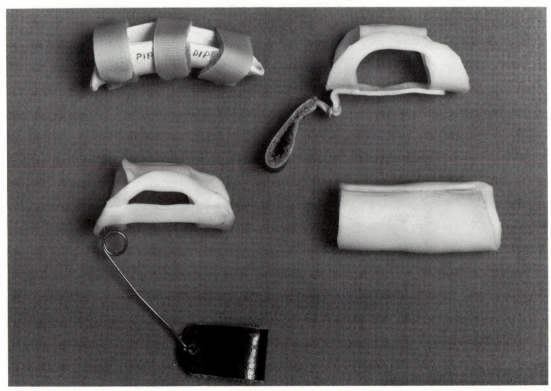

Figure 34–1

BOUTONNIERE DEFORMITY

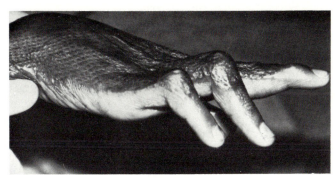

Figure 34-2

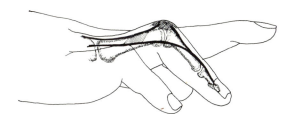

Figure 34-3

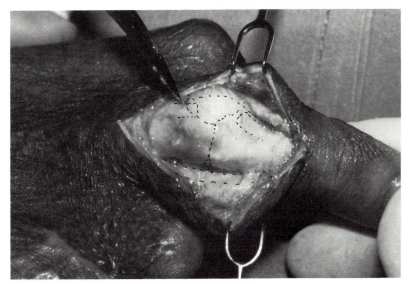

Figure 34-4

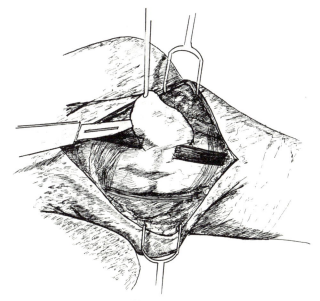

Figure 34-5

Figure 34-6. A 4-0 monofilament, horizontal, mattress suture is inserted in the proximal central tendon and continued through the cuff of scarred central slip near its insertion. The suture is tied with the proximal interphalangeal joint held in 10 to 15 degrees of flexion, to prevent too much shortening of the collateral ligament, which would compromise future flexion of the proximal interphalangeal joint.

Figure 34-7A, B. The transverse retinacular ligaments are incised on both sides of the finger, allowing the lateral bands to migrate to a more normal dorsal position. Some 5-0 monofilament sutures (usually two) unite the lateral bands distally to reconstruct the disrupted triangular ligament, while maintaining a space distal to the central tendon insertion.

Although some surgeons rely on a dressing to maintain the finger in proper position, it is helpful to insert a Kirschner wire across the proximal interphalangeal joint, maintaining it in 10 to 15 degrees' flexion, to reduce the chance of movement disrupting the ligament and tendon repairs. Wire fixation is maintained for four weeks postoperatively, when it is removed, and passive and active flexion and extension exercises are begun.

Figure 34-8A, B. Eight months postoperatively a reasonable result, with flexion and extension, is shown.

Pitfalls and Solutions

1. Ill-advised attempts at splinting that feature dorsal pressure may cause sloughing of soft tissue, down to and including the extensor tendon. Splints must be removed several times daily, and the skin observed for early signs of ulceration.

2. Do not suture the lateral bands to the central slip before determining the passive range of motion of the joint. Finger flexion will be impossible if lateral band repair is too distal and tight. Following repair, passive range of motion should be checked once again to ensure that too much tenodesis effect has not been created by returning the lateral bands dorsally.

3. If 45 degrees of proximal interphalangeal joint flexion is impossible, the lateral bands have been placed too far dorsally, or the repaired central slip is too short and tight. Correction must be made at this time.

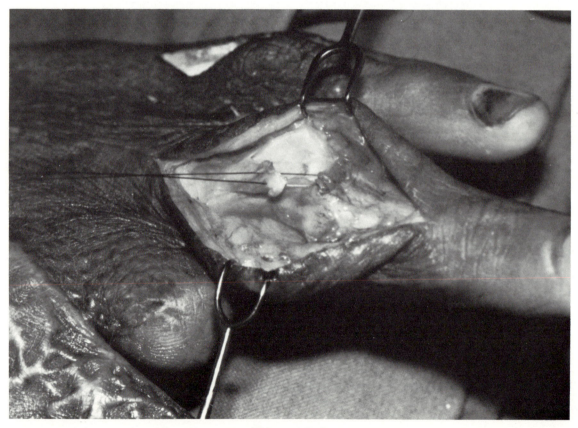

Figure 34-6

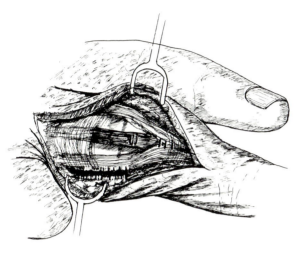

Figure 34-7A

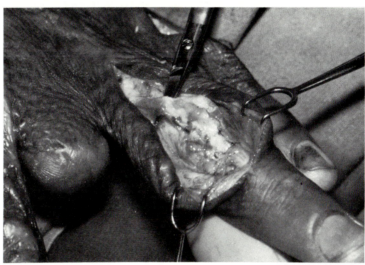

Figure 34-7B

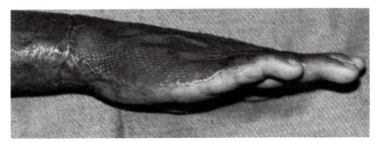

Figure 34-8A

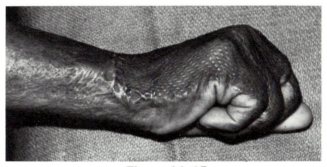

Figure 34-8B

35

Adduction Contracture of the Thumb

The Problem

Figures 35–1, 35–2, 35–3. Adduction contracture of the thumb following deep injury of the thumb web space is often associated with tethering of the thumb in extension. The mobility of the normal metacarpophalangeal joint of the thumb often leads to hyperextension of this joint when unyielding scar and contractures are interposed in the thumb and index metacarpal area. The result is adduction of the thumb, contracture of the first web space, and a pseudo-Froment's sign (hyperextension of the thumb metacarpophalangeal joint with flexion of the distal joint of the thumb). In this position, grasp is limited severely and normal pinch is obviated. Pulp-to-pulp apposition of the thumb and index or other digits becomes impossible, although side-to-side or "key" pinch remains.

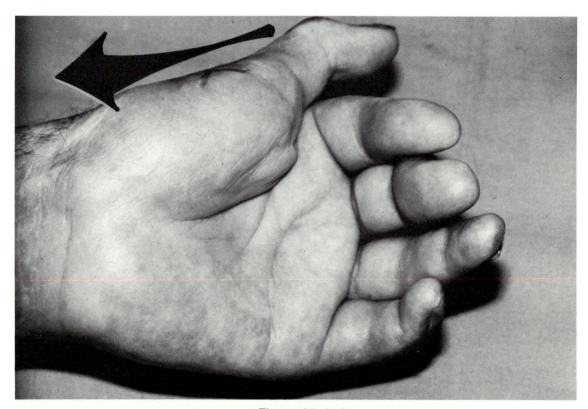

Figure 35–1

ADDUCTION CONTRACTURE OF THE THUMB

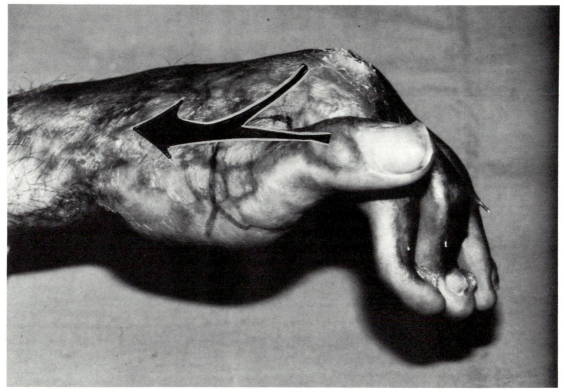

Figure 35-2

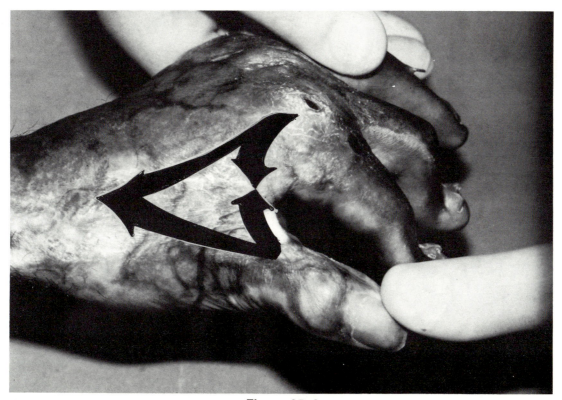

Figure 35-3

Technique

Figure 35–4. The incision of choice is transverse, and extends through the web space and over the metacarpophalangeal joint of the thumb. One must avoid injury to branches of the radial nerve supplying sensibility to this area by means of observation and cautious dissection in the subcutaneous space.

Figure 35–5. The fascia investing the adductor pollicis muscle usually is heavily scarred and must be incised widely. In the thicker areas, excision of this fascia is required. Occasionally, the tendinous insertion of the adductor pollicis muscle must be partially divided subperiosteally and allowed to retract. If complete division is required, the tendon may be sutured slightly proximal to the original insertion.

Figure 35–6. A Kirschner fixation wire is placed between the thumb and index metacarpals, with the thumb held in wide abduction. Fasciectomy of the lateral head of the first dorsal interosseous muscle, with further resection of the volar adductor pollicis fascia, is carried out as required. Great care must be taken to avoid injury to digital nerves to the thumb that lie superficially over the fascia and in the subcutaneous space in this area. Similarly, injury to the radial digital nerve to the index finger must be avoided because of its proximity to the distal part of the thumb web space. The metacarpophalangeal joint of the thumb is maintained in 30 degrees of flexion by means of a Kirschner wire. Release of the dorsal extensor mechanism overlying this joint may be necessary to further allow the distal phalanx to assume a neutral or slightly extended position.

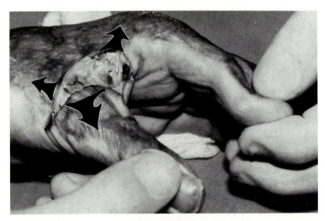

Figure 35–4

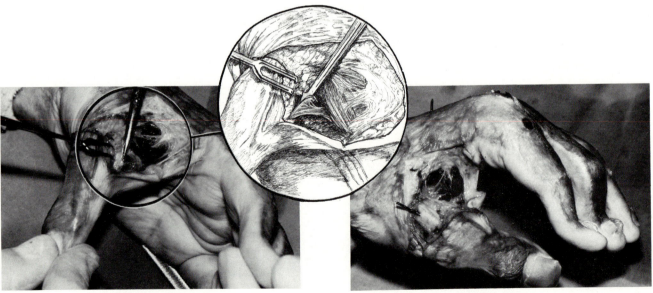

Figure 35–5   Figure 35–6

Figure 35–7. With the structures maintained in position, a split-thickness skin graft (0.014 to 0.016 inches) is applied to the large defect. Ten to 12 days postoperatively a dynamic splint is applied that allows wrist extension and flexion, maintenance of thumb metacarpal abduction, and metacarpophalangeal flexion. A static conformer in the first web space is used for several weeks. For the patient illustrated, the web space device included an extension to promote flexion of the distal phalanx of the index finger.

Figures 35–8, 35–9. The appropriate position for the thumb metacarpophalangeal joint, and for the patient's ability to oppose the pulp surfaces of this thumb and the digits, was achieved. Occasionally, lengthening of the extensor pollicis longus, extensor pollicis brevis, or abductor pollicis longus tendon(s) is required. Arthrodesis of the metacarpophalangeal joint is rarely necessary, but must be done in the event of deep destruction of the dorsal extensor mechanism.

Pitfalls and Solutions

1. Avoid sensory radial nerve branch injury through the transverse thumb incision by cautious dissection in the dorsal subcutaneous space.

2. Complete adductor pollicis fascial release must be done, but injury to the digital nerve to the thumb and index finger must be avoided.

3. Inadequate release of adductor fascia on both its doral and volar surfaces will lead to a recurrence of the contracture and hyperadduction of the thumb.

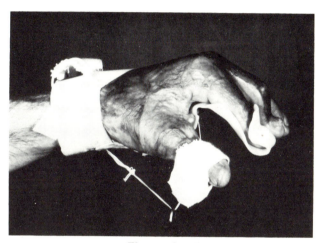

Figure 35–7

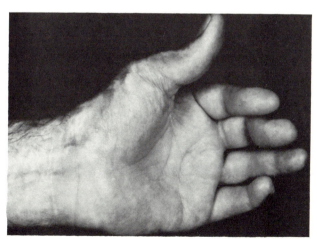

Figure 35–8

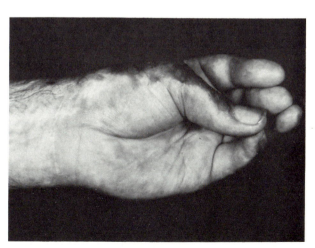

Figure 35–9

36

Scarring of Dorsal Thumb Web Skin: Anatomical Considerations

The Problem

Occasionally, local dorsal scarring of the thumb web skin occurs without significant injury to the leading edge of the web. Adduction contracture of the thumb does not take place, but excision of an irritated and painful scar is often requested by the patient.

Figure 36–1. A localized scar of the dorsal thumb web is seen. The patient complained of pain on abduction of the thumb and when holding large objects. The purpose of presenting this case is to emphasize an anatomical warning. Regardless of the technique chosen for repair, the ulnar neurovascular bundle of the thumb and radial digital nerve and artery of the index finger are in jeopardy of being cut inadvertently. Thus, one must not substitute a major problem for a minor one.

Technique

Figure 36–2. The scar is excised, and only minimal contracture was present.

Figure 36–3A, B. Advancement flaps are outlined on the dorsum and palmar surface of the thumb web. Thus, three local advancement flaps are generated, two from the proximal and distal volar aspect of the thumb web, and one from the central dorsal aspect. The flaps are dissected subcutaneously and undermined widely, care being taken to avoid any injury to underlying sensory nerves to the dorsum of the hand or index finger and thumb. Using blunt-tipped scissors, longitudinal dissection is performed along the course of the digital nerves. When sufficient soft tissue is under both flaps, dissection is extended toward their bases. Before the flaps are transposed, the nerves should be visualized and the surgeon assured they are intact.

Figures 36–4, 36–5. The flaps are sutured in position, creating a W-shaped incision that has completely altered the line of tension. The central point of the leading edge of the thumb web is unaltered, and wide-based, volar advancement flaps are interposed from the central point, proximally and distally. The normal, curved configuration of the uninjured leading edge of the thumb web is maintained.

Pitfalls and Solutions

1. Insufficient planning and size of the dorsal and volar flaps will lead to inadequate maintenance of a normal thumb-index web.

2. Injury to the nerves to the thumb and index finger and to those supplying sensation to the dorsum of the thumb web must be avoided by careful, subcutaneous dissection.

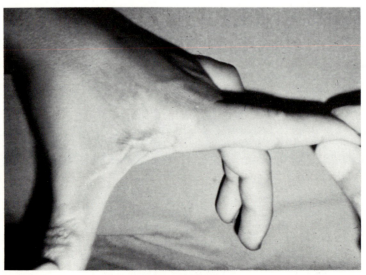

Figure 36–1

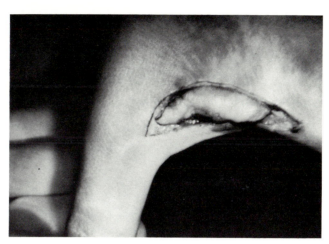

Figure 36-2

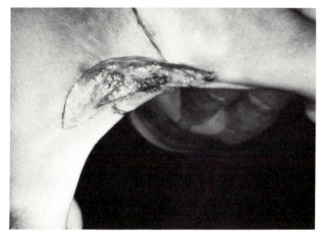

Figure 36-3A

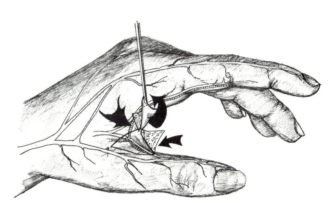

Figure 36-3B

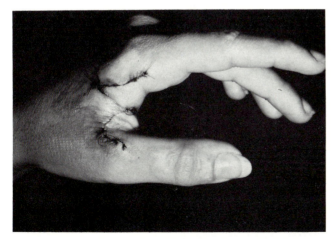

Figure 36-4

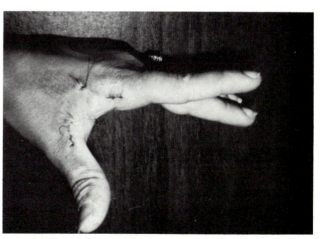

Figure 36-5

173

37

Pollicization

The Problem

Complex procedures such as pollicization of a digit to create a thumb are rarely required in burn injuries. However, in some patients who have had a devastating electrical injury, a high priority is placed upon improving useful function of a remaining hand.

Figures 37–1, 37–2. This patient suffered a severe electrical burn resulting in the loss of one arm and of the thumb on the contralateral hand. Pollicization after initial healing was elected, to restore pinch and grasp for this remaining hand.

Figure 37–3. Because the injury was very proximal, destroying the entire first metacarpal and a portion of the greater multangular bone, nearly all of the index digit distal to the metacarpophalangeal joint was required for adequate length.

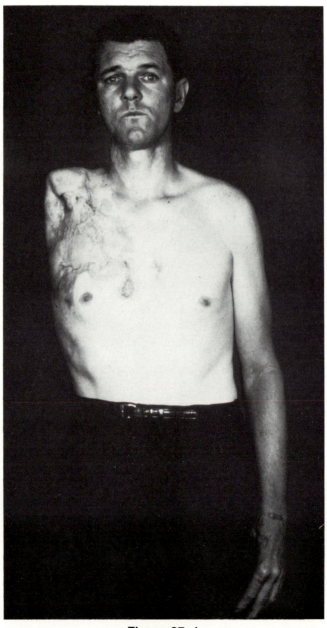

Figure 37–1

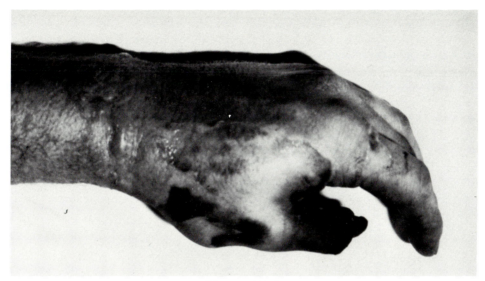

Figure 37-2

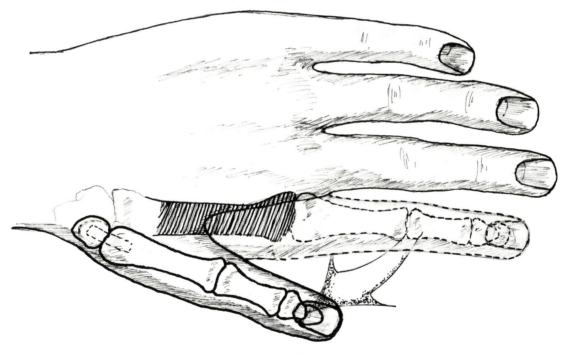

Figure 37-3

UPPER EXTREMITY

Technique

Figure 37–4. Incisions are planned at the base of the index digit overlying the index metacarpal, so that a circular incision is avoided. The tapered, roughly diamond-shaped incision will heal with less contracture than a circular one. A similar incision over the existing residual base of the thumb (in this case, a portion of the greater multangular bone) is made to allow accurate insetting of the transposed digit. A pneumatic tourniquet is used during surgery.

Figure 37–5. After debridement of the thumb, skin grafting was used for initial healing. The injury had resulted in destruction of the first web space and soft tissues radial to the index metacarpal. The skin graft was excised, revealing no radial neurovascular pedicle to the index digit.

Figure 37–6. The metacarpal was excised just distal to the proximal flaring of the metacarpal base, care being taken not to injure the common digital artery and nerve to the index digit. This is best accomplished by removing the metacarpal subperiosteally throughout its length. The extensor and flexor tendons to the digit are isolated and preserved.

Figure 37–7. Transection of the proximal phalanx of the index digit at a level predetermined to allow pinch against the long, ring, and small digits is done with a high-speed, air-driven saw. The digital nerve and artery remaining on the ulnar side of the digit are carefully guarded during transection of the phalanx. Separation of the common digital nerve to the adjacent sides of the index and middle digits is required to allow adequate proximal positioning of the index finger. This is done under magnification with gentle, blunt dissection, which separates the perineurium over the proper digital nerves at the bifurcation of the common digital nerve. After identification of the extensor and flexor tendons, and the neurovascular pedicle to the digit, and remaining capsular attachments on the ulnar surface are divided, and the index digit isolated on its neurovascular and tendinous pedicle. In this case the residual greater multangular bone is exposed and cleared of fibrous tissue, and a maximal surface area is made with a dental burr.

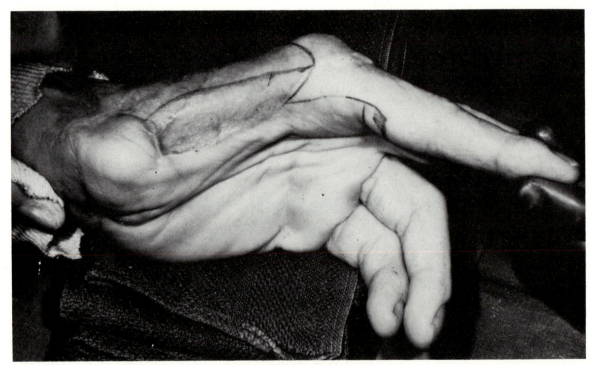

Figure 37–4

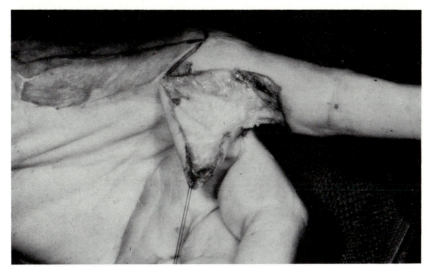

Figure 37-5

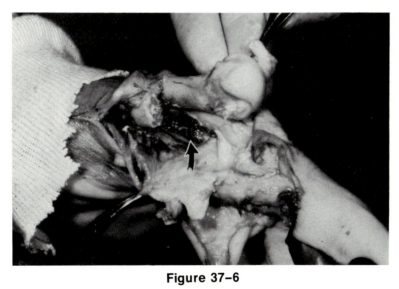

Figure 37-6

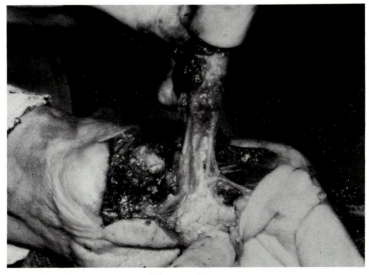

Figure 37-7

Figure 37–8. The isolated index digit is tested for apposition with the prepared recipient site on the surface of the greater multangular bone. Adjustment of the surface of the index proximal phalanx and the greater multangular is made with the dental burr to provide maximal bone-to-bone apposition.

Figure 37–9A. A small bone peg is fashioned from the resected portion of the index metacarpal, and machined with a dental burr to approximately 1.5 cm in length and 4 to 5 mm in diameter. Using a 4- to 5-mm drill, a socket is made in the greater multangular bone, 0.75 cm deep. A similar socket is drilled into the proximal phalanx of the index digit. The tourniquet is released and hemostasis achieved. The vascularity of the index digit is assessed, and if the tourniquet time has reached one hour, 15 to 20 minutes must pass before one can be certain of adequate circulation to the digit. During this wait, further assessment and establishment of hemostasis is accomplished, as hematoma will lead to compression of the vascular pedicle and necrosis of the transposed digit.

B. The index digit is placed on the bone peg seated into the greater multangular socket. The digit is rotated so that passive pulp-to-pulp apposition between it and the middle, ring, and small digits is achieved. When this adjustment is final, a single Kirschner wire is driven through the proximal interphalangeal joint of the index, across the fusion site, and into the distal radius for fixation.

Figure 37–10. The index digit should lie as if it were an extension of the radius. Since the radial surface of the index metacarpal was destroyed in the initial injury, medium-thickness (0.014- to 0.018-inch) split skin grafts are used to resurface this area. An occlusive dressing with plaster splints incorporated into it is applied for protection of the graft and transposed digit. The extremity is kept elevated, and circulation to the index digit is observed frequently during the postoperative period. In this patient, no adjustment of extensor or flexor tendon length was required because of the long segment of index digit used. In patients with portions of the thumb metacarpal remaining, however, the arc of rotation of the index digit is such that the extensor tendon must be shortened to produce an effective amplitude. In these cases, incisions are made over the distal wrist after the transposed digit is fixed into position. By exposure and retraction of the index extensor tendons and flexors, superficialis and profundus, the amount of shortening that produces pulp-to-pulp apposition of the index to the other digits is assessed. The respective tendons are not divided in this maneuver, but rather the slack is taken up by suturing the tendons to themselves in the shortened position.

Fourteen to 18 weeks of immobilization are required to achieve solid osteosynthesis at the fusion site. During this time, however, passive range of motion and active flexion and extension of the distal joint of the index finger are allowed with supervision. These movements are done in a protective splint after an initial healing period of four weeks.

Figures 37–11, 37–12. Four months after pollicization of the damaged index digit, the "thumb" appears somewhat long owing to the absence of a thenar eminence. Grasp and pinch functions are restored.

Pitfalls and Solutions

1. Patients must be selected carefully, being those with severely compromised hands. They must be motivated and able to participate in a long course of hand rehabilitation.

2. Injury to the neurovascular supply to the donor digit is the commonest problem preventing a successful result. An intimate knowledge of the anatomy and technique of dissection is required to avoid this danger.

3. The length of donor digit must be determined preoperatively, with the goal of pulp-to-pulp apposition of the new thumb to the remaining fingers. In burned patients the functional result is prime, and the esthetic result that frequently is possible in congenital or other traumatic losses of the thumb is not often achieved.

4. The pitfalls in this complex operation are many. The work of Littler and Chase should be reviewed by those contemplating carrying out this reconstruction.

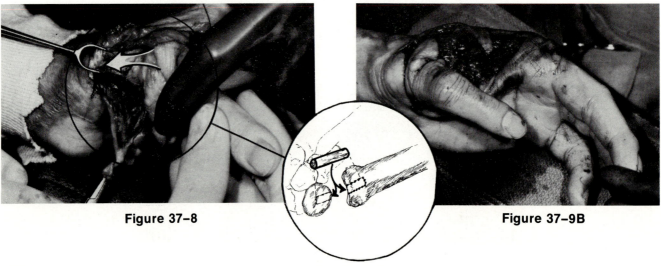

Figure 37–8

Figure 37–9A

Figure 37–9B

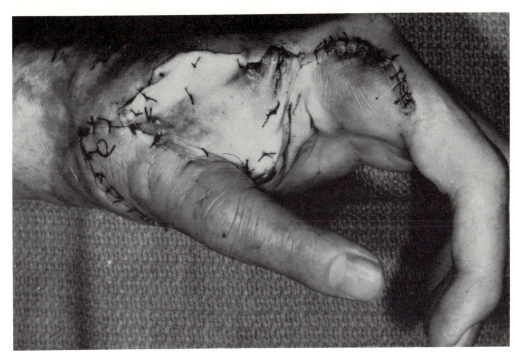

Figure 37–10

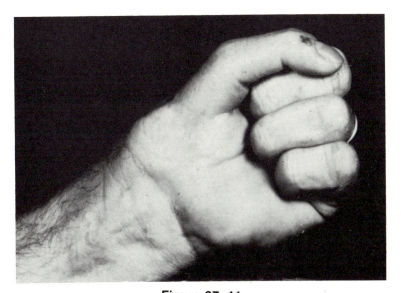

Figure 37–11

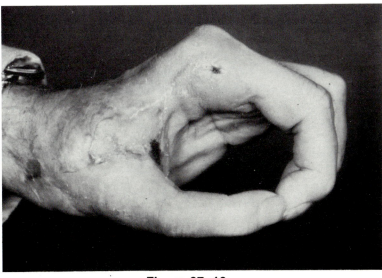

Figure 37–12

Burn Syndactyly: The "Hourglass" Procedure

The Problem

Burn syndactyly is a condition in which one or both of the following anatomical derangements are noted:

a. The subjacent sides of digits are wounded, resulting in actual healing together of the digits, with destruction of the interdigital web.

b. There is palmar burn injury that leads to distal distraction of the interdigital web.

Burn syndactyly is thus distinguished from dorsal adduction contractures of the digits, a condition in which the interdigital web is usually intact and in a normal position.

Technique

The repair of true burn syndactyly is based on a procedure used for the reconstruction of congenital syndactyly described by Bevin in 1973, and referred to as the "hourglass" procedure. The operative reconstruction utilizes a dorsal pedicle flap of healed, remodeled, burned skin that is designed with the anatomy of the digits and their webs in mind. The flap is planned so that resultant incisions will not lead to linear contractures across the web itself. The normal anatomy of the position and contour of interdigital webs is remarkably constant. By relying on this constant finding, and relating this to easily determined landmarks, satisfactory reconstruction of burn syndactyly is achieved. Patients are chosen for reconstruction only after sufficient time from their injury has passed so that the dorsal skin or previously grafted skin is mature, pliable, and fully healed. Hourglass pedicle flaps have been uniformly viable under these conditions.

Figure 38–1. The distal volar leading edge of a normal web lies one-half of the distance from the axis of rotation of the metacarpophalangeal joint and the axis of rotation of the proximal interphalangeal joint. A point one-half of the distance between the leading edge of the interdigital web and the axis of rotation of the metacarpophalangeal joint marks the distal extent of the lumbrical canal and its dorsal and volar fascia. Using a dorsally and proximally based pedicle flap, its central portion must be narrower than the proximal or distal width so that the flap will conform to the underlying anatomy, and avoid any incision that crosses the surface of the new interdigital web. The narrow portion of the flap must lie at a point one-half of the distance between the distal extent of the lumbrical canal and the distal volar leading edge of the web. The pedicle flap must be of sufficient length to create both the dorsal surface and length of the new web, to fold upon itself, and to insert into the distal volar surface of the palm. The width of the distal margin of the hourglass pedicle flap is equal to the distance between the mid-dorsal planes of the adjacent digits.

The landmarks and anatomical considerations are summarized as follows (Fig. 38–1):

1. The axis of rotation of the interphalangeal joint.

2. The axis of rotation of the metacarpophalangeal joint.

3. The normal position of the distal volar leading edge of the interdigital web (one-half of the distance between 1 and 2).

4. The distal extent of the lumbrical canal and its dorsal and volar fascia (one-half of the distance between 2 and 3).

5. The narrow portion, or "waist," of the dorsal pedicle flap (one-half of the distance between 3 and 4).

6. The distal margin of the dorsal pedicle flap (one-half of the distance between 1 and 3).

7. The width of the distal margin is taken as the distance between the mid-dorsal planes of the adjacent digits.

These points are marked in the operating room with Brilliant Green solution on the tip of a fine needle, and a flap is drawn as indicated, yielding an hourglass-shaped dorsal pedicle flap that is based proximally. The flap is dissected from distal to proximal, preserving a 1- to 2-mm thickness of subcutaneous fat on the undersurface. Proximal dissection is halted at a point just proximal to the level of the lumbrical canal fascia, which is carefully preserved. The palmar surface, whether it is normal skin or healed, mature burn scar, is divided in the midline between the adjacent digits proximally to the level of the volar lumbrical canal fascia. Distal to the level of the proximal interphalangeal joints, any adherence of adjacent digits is usually separated by mirror-image, Z-shaped incisions that create triangular flaps used to resurface the distal portion of the digits.

BURN SYNDACTYLY: THE "HOURGLASS" PROCEDURE

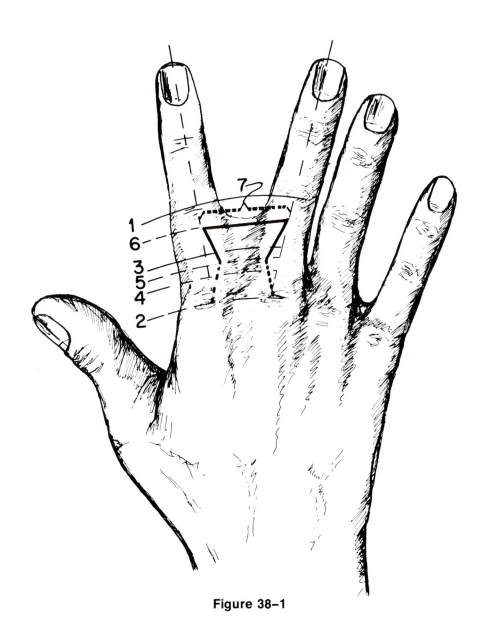

Figure 38–1

Figure 38-2. After the hourglass flap is raised, skin defects, usually quite rectangular in shape, will result on the subjacent sides of the involved digits. The flap is folded volarly, and a trapezoid of normal, distal palmar skin or healed burn scar (as the case may be) in that area is excised. This trapezoid is the exact shape of the distal portion of the pedicle flap. The flap is sutured into the trapezoidal volar defect with nonabsorbable sutures. The rectangular wounds resulting on the subjacent sides of the digits are resurfaced with full-thickness skin grafts taken from a groin crease, and are sutured into the defects with nonabsorbable sutures. The groin donor site is closed with absorbable, subcuticular sutures and a continuous, nonabsorbable intradermal suture, which is removed two weeks postoperatively. The hand is dressed with the digits in slight abduction, and with the small joints in 30 to 45 degrees of flexion. Nonadherent, antiseptic gauze is placed over the suture lines, and a single layer of coarse meshed gauze between the fingers. A bolus of fluffed gauze or mechanics' waste is used to maintain the position of the digits and the transverse palmar arch. A short-arm occlusive dressing is applied and secured with adhesive strips. A volar plaster splint may be incorporated into the dressing for additional support and immobilization if desired.

Figures 38-3, 38-4. This patient sustained a palmar burn 20 years previously. Primary healing had occurred, resulting in distal distraction of the interdigital web to the level of the proximal interphalangeal joints of the index and long digits.

Figure 38-5. At operation, an hourglass flap has been dissected as described, and sutured into position. Based on its dorsal, proximal attachment, the flap has been folded upon itself and inserted into the distal palm.

Figure 38-6. The wounds on the subjacent sides of the digits have been resurfaced with full-thickness skin grafts taken from the groin crease.

Figure 38-7. The same patient, six years postoperatively, is seen with the index-long digit interdigital web reconstructed. The reconstructed web of the right hand (*a*) is compared with the patient's normal left index-long digit interdigital web (*b*).

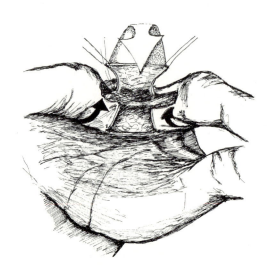

Figure 38-2

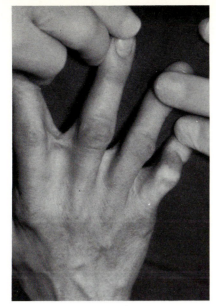

Figure 38-3

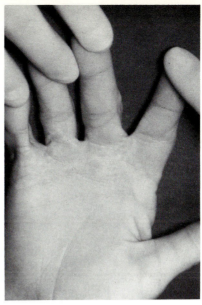

Figure 38-4

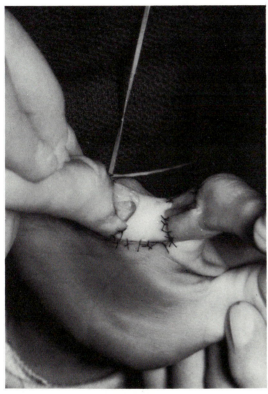

Figure 38-5

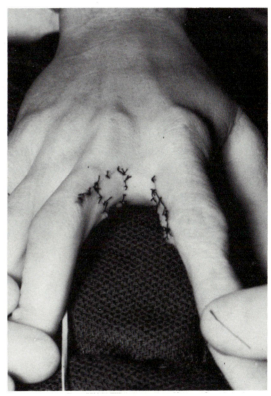

Figure 38-6

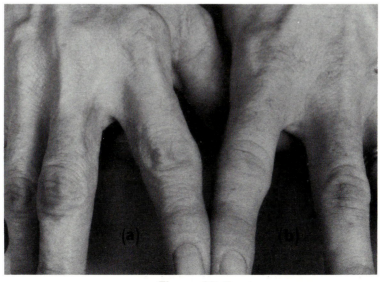

Figure 38-7

183

Figure 38-8. The same normal and operative landmarks are used in the situation in which digits are conjoined after healing of burns, and the interdigital webs have been destroyed. This child developed burn syndactyly of all four digits. There was destruction of the interdigital webs in addition to healing of the digits to one another.

The various landmarks are marked at surgery to create a dorsal, hourglass pedicle flap for reconstruction of the webs. In this patient the index-long digit and the ring-small digit interdigital webs were reconstructed in one procedure, leaving the long-ring web for a second operation. Generally, immediately adjacent web reconstructions are not done in one operation for fear of disrupting too much of the venous circulation of the flaps and the dorsal structures at the bases of the digits.

Figure 38-9. At the completion of the initial operative procedure, the hourglass flaps are in position, and the skin defects on the subjacent sides of the digits are resurfaced with full-thickness skin grafts taken from the groin crease. Distal to the proximal interphalangeal joints, flaps from adjacent digits were used to resurface the areas resulting from distal separation of the extensive syndactyly.

Figure 38-10. The same patient's hand is seen four years after reconstruction of all the interdigital webs in two operative procedures. Closer views show the three interdigital webs and the appropriate appearance of the space between the digits.

When the burn injury has been significant enough to produce burn syndactyly as described, several months to over a year are required for adequate softening and pliability of the injured healed skin to be achieved prior to reconstruction. Pressure garments, massage, and maintenance of hygiene are mandatory in assisting this process. Under these conditions, and with careful dissection after considering the landmarks as described, this flap is well vascularized with arterial and venous vessels. The flap is durable, and produces an excellent functional and esthetic result that persists over time.

Pitfalls and Solutions

1. The landmarks, both anatomical and surgical, must be studied and marked accurately. Brilliant Green solution tattooed with a fine needle must be used to avoid obliteration of the marks during surgery.

2. Preservation of digital neurovascular structures is critical, and dissection is carried out with tourniquet control.

3. Preservation of the dorsal and volar layers of the distal fascial extent of the lumbrical canal is required. Failure to do this will result in a V-shaped web space, and a too proximal final position of the leading edge of the interdigital web.

4. The correct diagnosis must be made. This reconstructive procedure is not indicated for dorsal adduction contractures that require a resurfacing procedure after release of the contracture, rather than a recreation of a new interdigital web as outlined for true burn syndactyly.

BURN SYNDACTYLY: THE "HOURGLASS" PROCEDURE

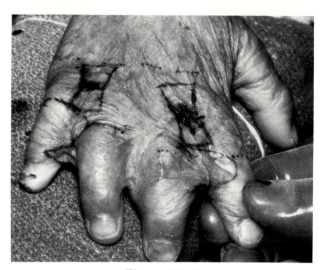

Figure 38-8

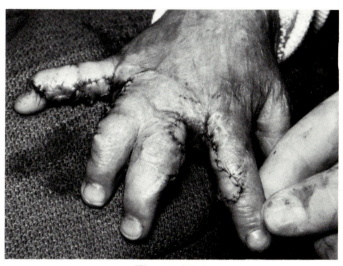

Figure 38-9

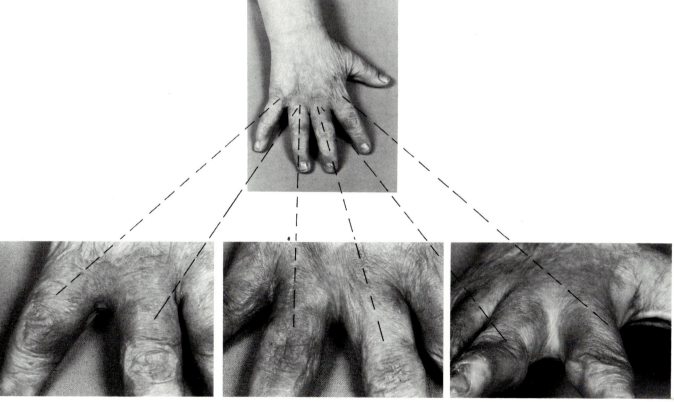

Figure 38-10

39

Dorsal Adduction Contractures of the Fingers

The Problem

Figures 39–1, 39–2. A hand is illustrated with the common finding of dorsal burn contractures between the thumb and index digit, and similar contractures involving the other fingers. The effect of this scarring is to pull the dorsal hand skin distally and create a dorsal "hood," with intact palmar interdigital web skin. This condition should *not* be referred to as "burn syndactyly," which is an unusual condition of absolute loss of skin on the lateral, adjacent surfaces of the digits with actual healing of these surfaces together. Also, in true burn syndactyly, palmar scar in the interdigital areas leads to distraction of the palmar skin distally, which is unusual in the presence of dorsal adduction contractures.

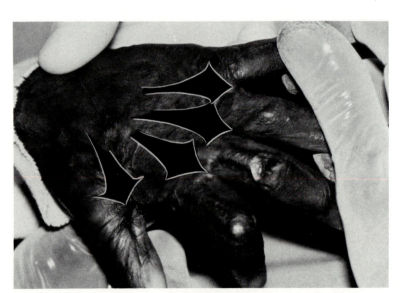

Figure 39–1

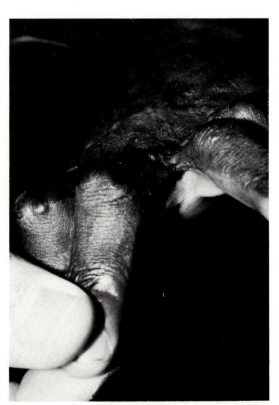

Figure 39–2

DORSAL ADDUCTION CONTRACTURES OF THE FINGERS

Technique

Figures 39–3, 39–4. The method of incision to release the various contractures, preserving the intact lateral digital skin and palmar interdigital webs, is illustrated. Excision of scar is not often required, but if the scar is deep and hypertrophic it is excised with care. Caution is required in the interdigital incisions and dissection to avoid injury to the rich venous plexus present in this area. Troublesome bleeding after release of the pneumatic tourniquet used in this procedure may result if these venous structures are disrupted. The incisions are carried deeply in the case of the thumb-index web; to expose and divide the fascia overlying the adductor pollicis and the first dorsal interosseous muscles. This will allow proximal retraction of the remainder of the dorsal skin, and full abduction of the thumb. Incision across the dorsal hooding scar of the digits is done similarly, with undermining of the entire dorsal intermetacarpal area. Adjacent intermetacarpal areas are not operated upon in one procedure because of the possibility of compromise of dorsal venous circulation, and because multiple interdigital dressings may lead to compression of the neurovascular structures to the digits. In the course of dissection the intermetacarpal ligaments are retained, and care is taken to avoid injury to digital nerves and vessels that may be displaced dorsally within the scar.

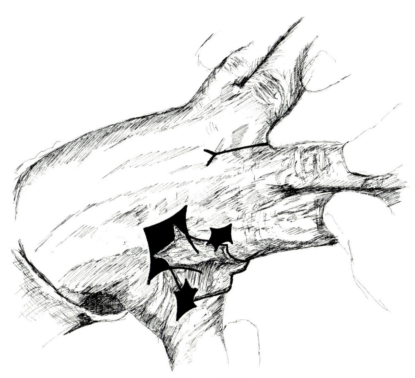

Figure 39–3

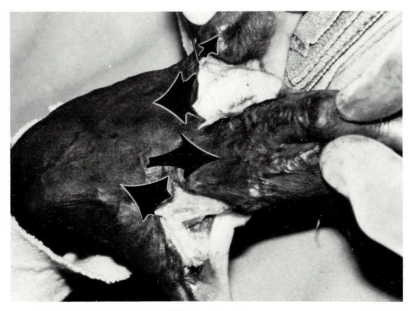

Figure 39–4

UPPER EXTREMITY

Figures 39–5, 39–6. After completing the releases, medium-thickness skin grafts (0.016-inch) are applied, with the digits fully abducted to insure adequate surface coverage. The monofilament sutures are cut short and not tied over bolsters in this area. Bolstered dressings in the interdigital area can often cause undue pressure on the lateral surfaces of the digits, interfering with their circulation. Instead, a carefully molded occlusive dressing of nonadherent gauze is placed on the grafts, followed by barely moistened gauze strips placed carefully between the digits; lastly, a bulky layer of mechanics' waste is added. This dressing may be complemented by external plaster splints for further immobilization. The extremity is maintained in elevation postoperatively for five to seven days, at which time the grafts and wounds are inspected.

Figure 39–7A, B. Following suture removal (as illustrated in another patient) and adequate healing of skin grafts, splinting is begun. Small tubes of foam rubber are placed within finger cots, and positioned vertically in the interdigital spaces. They are held in place with a compressive glove intermittently for several months, to maintain the gains in abduction achieved at operation.

Pitfalls and Solutions

1. After incision of the interdigital web scar, longitudinal dissection must be used to avoid injury to digital neurovascular structures that may be displaced dorsally in this area. Indiscriminate transverse dissection may disrupt these structures.

2. Injury to the dorsal venous plexus must be avoided. Hemostasis is achieved after release of the tourniquet and before application of skin grafts, to avoid hematoma and necrosis of the grafts.

3. The digits must be maintained in abduction with soft, interdigital splints that should be worn for several months.

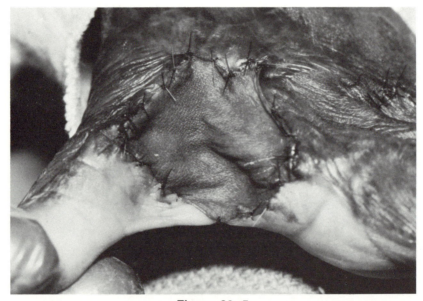

Figure 39–5

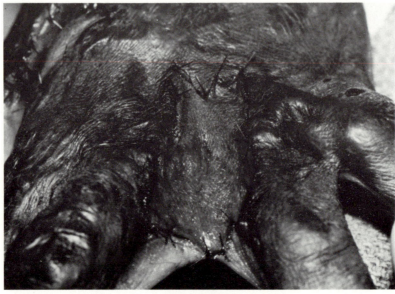

Figure 39–6

DORSAL ADDUCTION CONTRACTURES OF THE FINGERS

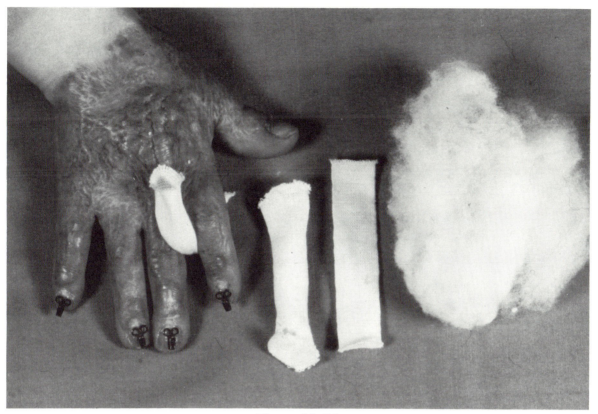

Figure 39–7A

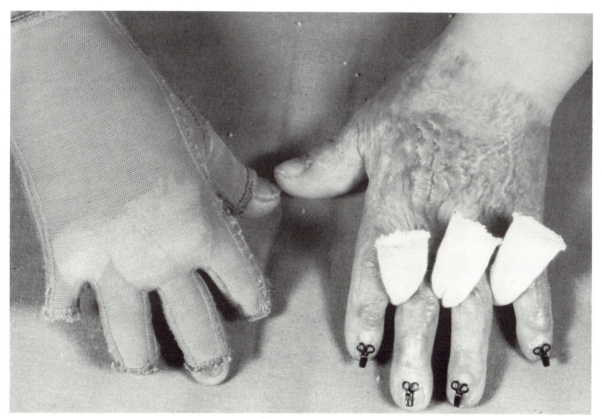

Figure 39–7B

40

Abduction Contracture of the Small Finger

The Problem

Fixed abduction of the small finger following a burn of the dorsum of the hand may reduce the functional breadth of the palm and power grasp, because the fingers cannot act in concert. Striking or "catching" the finger on objects is also a hazard. The deformity may result from:

a. A dorsal, lateral, linear scar contracture.

b. Ischemic contracture of the abductor digiti quinti minimi muscle secondary to a circumferential burn with marked edema that compromises the muscle blood flow.

c. A combination of a and b, which may produce ulnar dislocation of the extensor tendon and shortening of the ulnar collateral ligament.

Technique

Figures 40–1, 40–2. A linear scar contracture, holding the small finger in fixed abduction, is illustrated. Although the contracture is linear, no Z-plasty or other local flaps are attempted because blood supply of the surrounding scar tissue is poor. A transverse incision is made across the scar at the metacarpophalangeal joint level.

ABDUCTION CONTRACTURE OF THE SMALL FINGER

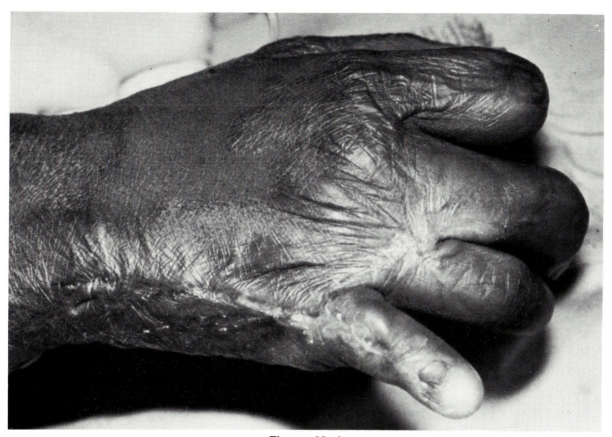

Figure 40-1

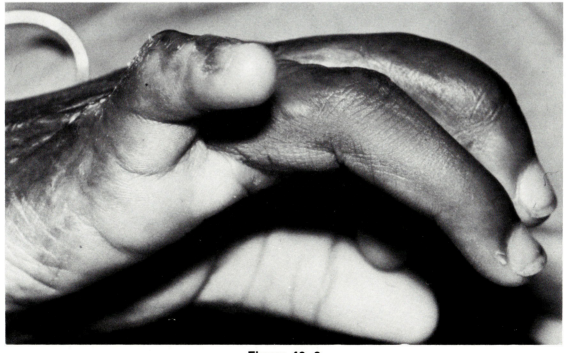

Figure 40-2

Figure 40–3A, B. Exposure of the hypothenar musculature revealed a fibrotic abductor muscle *(arrow)*, which was cut at its tendinous insertion and allowed to retract proximally. Because of the chronic ulnar deviation, the ulnar collateral ligament was shortened, and it is partially incised until the finger can be brought into neutral or radial deviation. A Kirschner wire is placed longitudinally, through the metacarpophalangeal joint, to hold the finger in its corrected position. This wire should be left in place for three weeks following surgery.

Figure 40–4. If ulnar dislocation of the extensor tendon has occurred, a longitudinal incision must be made through the radial aspect *(a,b)* of the extensor mechanism at the metacarpophalangeal joint level. The central slip of the extensor is then repaired in a "vest over pants" *(c,d)* fashion over the axis of the joint, after a relaxing incision is made along the ulnar aspect of the extensor mechanism *(c)*.

Figures 40–5, 40–6. The skin defect is closed with a split-thickness graft, and one year later the patient was able to fully abduct and adduct the finger.

Pitfalls and Solutions

1. Failure to recognize ulnar dislocation of the extensor tendon as a contributing cause of the abductor deformity will lead to an incomplete correction.

2. Failure to incise the ulnar collateral ligament and pin the finger in the corrected position will lead to a recurrent deformity.

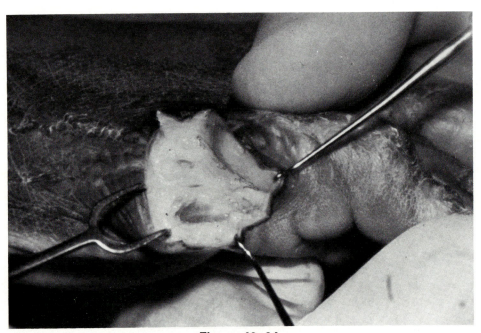

Figure 40–3A

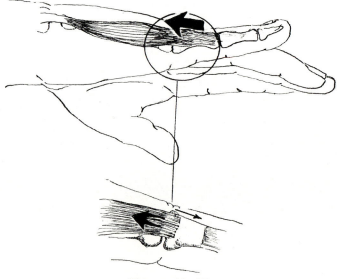

Figure 40–3B

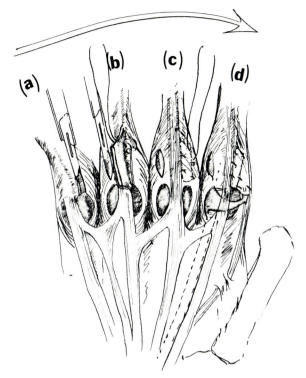

Figure 40-4

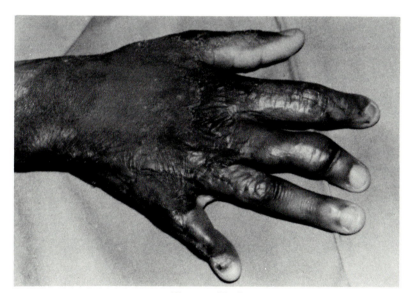

Figure 40-5

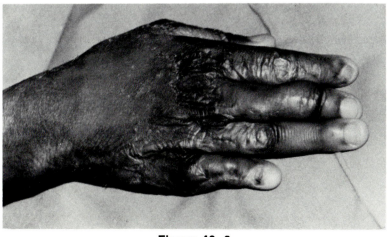

Figure 40-6

Trunk, Genitalia, and Lower Extremity

41

Caudal Contracture of the Breast

The Problem

When severe scar contracture has produced a caudal displacement of the breast, the result is marked asymmetry and restriction of contour. This injury may occur before puberty and lead to interference with normal breast development. Reconstruction is planned to reposition the breast and restore symmetry of the inframammary folds as esthetically as possible.

Figures 41–1, 41–2, 41–3. A patient aged nine had been burned at age two. The wounds healed without skin grafting, but marked caudal displacement of the breast occurred as the child grew.

Technique

Figure 41–2. If a normal contralateral breast is present, the following measurements are made:

a. The distance from the midclavicle to the nipple;

b. The distance from the margin of the areola to the inframammary fold of that breast;

and the following landmarks are noted:

c. The inframammary fold should lie on a line through the midhumerus projected across the chest wall;

d. The distance from the inferior edge of the areola to the inframammary fold is usually 5 to 6 cm. The inframammary fold of the displaced breast is marked with respect to the normal breast.

CAUDAL CONTRACTURE OF THE BREAST

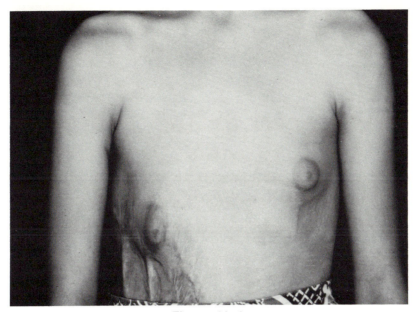

Figure 41-1

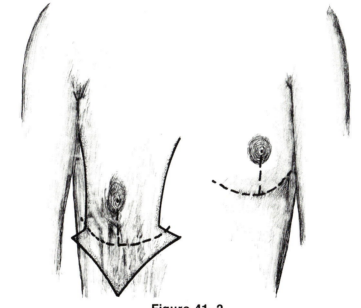

Figure 41-2

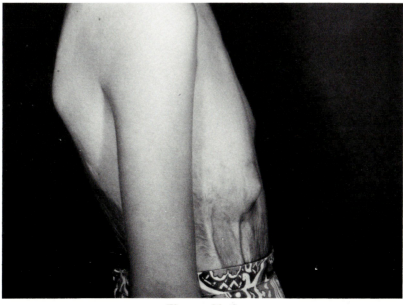

Figure 41-3

197

Figures 41–4, 41–5. Incision alone, carried to the rectus abdominis fascia, usually results in release of the breast superiorly. Elevation is further enhanced by undermining the breast at the level of the rectus abdominis fascia and on the pectoralis major fascia superiorly as the breast is repositioned upward. The incision made in the inframammary fold must be carried laterally enough to insure restoration of the lateral contour of the breast. One should avoid incision medially over the sternum because of the common complication of hypertrophic scarring in this area. If distal contracture remains over the abdominal wall, undermining of that area on the rectus abdominis fascia is performed.

The arm is fully abducted at the shoulder to make certain that adequate upward positioning of the breast has been achieved, and that the resulting wound is not resurfaced with too small a skin graft.

Figure 41–6. Medium-thickness skin grafts (0.014 to 0.018 inches) are sutured into place. The resulting wounds in these cases often are very large, requiring several hundred square centimeters of skin graft. In order to maintain the restored position of the breast, the skin grafts are dressed with nonadherent gauze, and a tie-over, bolstered, occlusive dressing is applied. The arm is splinted in abduction using plaster or heat-labile, plastic material that is applied in the operating room over the dressing. The splinted position of the arm is maintained for seven to ten days until graft healing is adequate. Range of motion exercises for the arm are begun at that time, and the abduction splint is worn during sleep for three or four weeks.

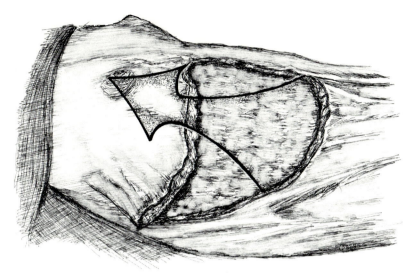
Figure 41-4

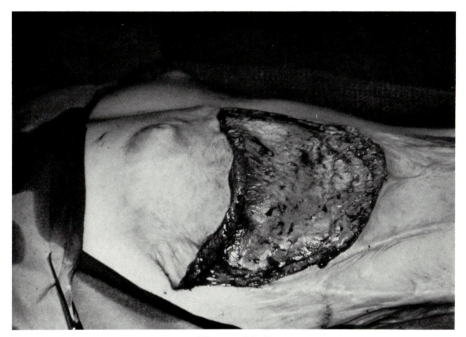
Figure 41-5

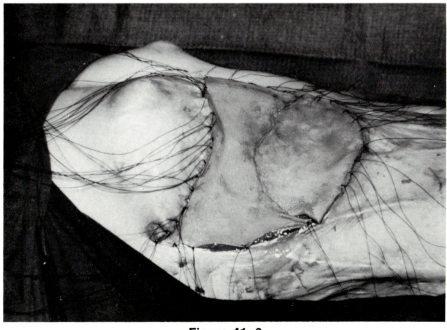
Figure 41-6

Figures 41–7, 41–8. The patient is seen five years later, at age 14, with good restoration of breast position and symmetry of the inframammary folds. Breast development is just beginning at this time.

Figure 41–9. The same patient at age 18, nine years after reconstructive surgery, has development of both breasts and acceptable symmetry. No reconstruction of the nipple or areola was indicated in this case.

In the event of destruction of the nipple-areola complex in the prepubescent patient, it is usually advisable to await puberty and final breast development before attempting reconstruction. In cases of unilateral loss of the nipple-areola complex without significant breast deformity, reconstruction can be done before puberty if the loss is a source of anguish to the patient.

Pitfalls and Solutions

1. Landmarks must be carefully determined and incisions marked prior to surgery, with the patient standing erect (especially in the event of bilateral breast deformity). Marking the incisions with the patient supine may result in gross asymmetry later.

2. Undermining is performed at the muscular fascial level to achieve adequate release. Injury to sensory nerves must be avoided if at all possible. Superiorly, dissection must be done at the level of the pectoralis fascia, or direct injury to breast tissue may result.

3. Skin grafting is done with the ipsilateral arm in abduction, to avoid too small a graft and the recurrence of caudal displacement of the breast.

CAUDAL CONTRACTURE OF THE BREAST

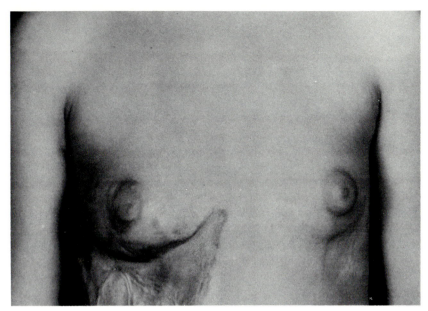

Figure 41-7

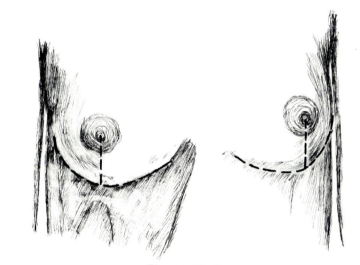

Figure 41-8

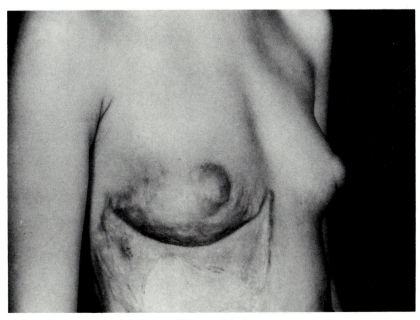

Figure 41-9

42

Lateral Contracture of the Breast

The Problem

Lateral contracture with displacement of the breast occurs more often than medial contracture, because burn injury to the axilla and lateral trunk is more frequent.

Figure 42–1A, B. In the event of lateral fixation, any concomitant axillary contractures should be corrected prior to reconstruction of the breast (as has been done in this patient). Thus, movement of the arm, and its effect upon normal elevation of the breast through the action of the pectoralis major muscle, will be improved before breast surgery.

Technique

Figure 42–2. A lateral contracture of the breast also shows obliteration of the lateral mammary fold and contour.

Figures 42–2, 42–3. The incision retains the attachment of the breast to the soft tissues of the chest wall at the inframammary and lateral mammary folds, but transects laterally the contracted skin and scar tissue that has displaced the breast. The inframammary fold should lie on a line crossing the midhumerus projected across the anterior chest.

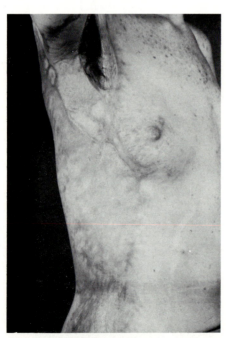

Figure 42–1A

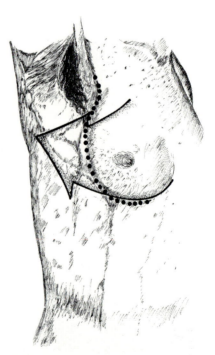

Figure 42–1B

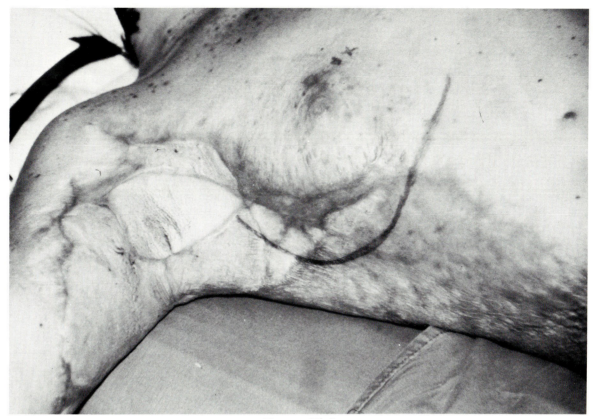

Figure 42-2

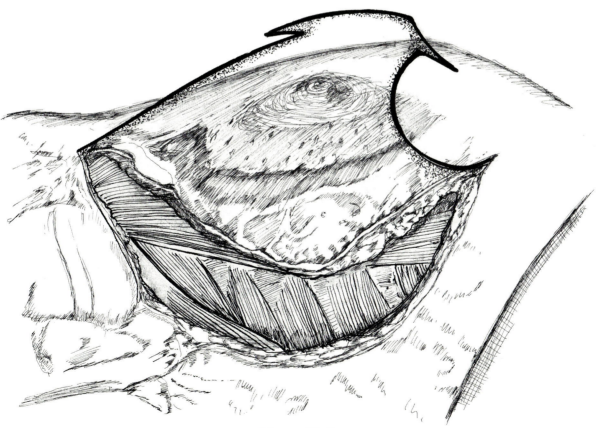

Figure 42-3

Figure 42-4. Laterally, dissection is performed at the level of the fascia overlying the latissimus dorsi muscle, and medially, just above the fascia over the pectoralis major muscle. Care is taken to avoid injury to the thoracodorsal nerve and other intercostobrachial nerves that lie in this region. The breast itself is undermined at the level of the pectoralis fascia if considerable relocation medially is required. The aim of this maneuver is to recreate the lateral mammary contour and insure separation of the breast soft tissue from the axilla.

The resulting wound surface area is maximized by placing the ipsilateral arm in extension and full abduction at the shoulder. Medium-thickness skin grafts (0.014- to 0.018-inch) are used to resurface this defect. After suture of the skin grafts into place, soft, bulky, occlusive dressings are applied so that the arm may be splinted in abduction at the shoulder. A molded splint of plaster or heat-labile, plastic material is constructed over the occlusive dressing in the operating room, to insure protection of the skin grafts and prevent wound contracture caused by adduction of the arm during healing.

Figures 42-5, 42-6. Postoperatively, with adduction of the arm, there is a sharp delineation below axilla and breast, and no lateral contracture. If the nipple-areola complex is disfigured or missing, its reconstruction is usually delayed until a second procedure. Attempts to resurface lateral defects, using high axillary skin out of the confine of the cupola of the axilla, are undesirable. Prosthetic implantation for restoration of deficient breast volume, if necessary, is also carried out at a later procedure. Symmetry with the other breast is easier to achieve after healing of the primary reconstruction.

In the prepubescent patient, release and resurfacing procedures only are done. Following puberty and development of both breasts, further surgery may be indicated to recreate symmetrical contours and volumes.

Pitfalls and Solutions

1. Injury to the sensory nerves coursing in the region of the axilla and lateral chest wall toward the breast tissue should be avoided.

2. After incision and/or excision of scar to release the breast, the surface area of the resultant wound must be maximized by abduction of the arm at the shoulder prior to skin grafting, or recurrence of the lateral displacement of the breast may ensue.

3. Postoperative splinting is maintained to avoid early adduction of the arm and possible foreshortening of the operative wound.

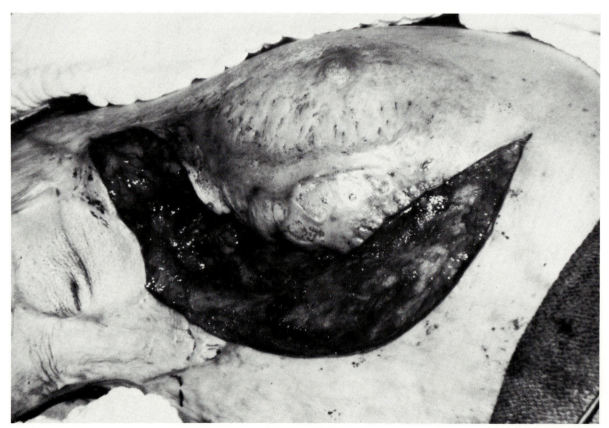

Figure 42-4

LATERAL CONTRACTURE OF THE BREAST

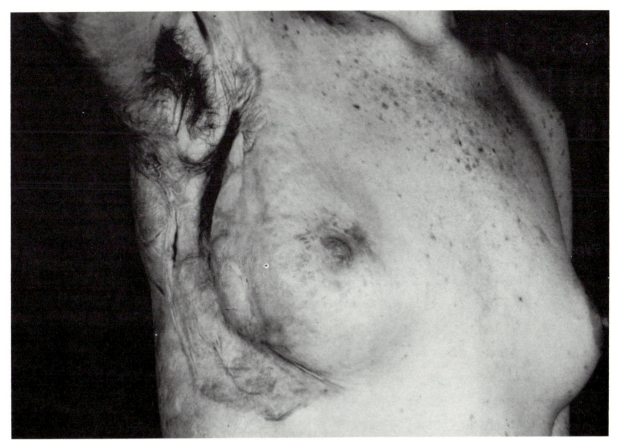

Figure 42–5

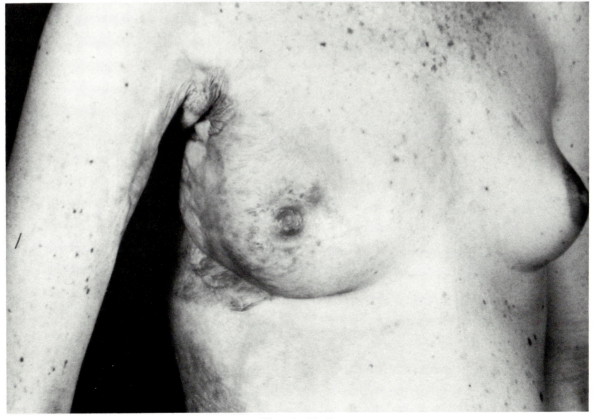

Figure 42–6

43

Loss of Breast Volume and Destruction of the Nipple-Areola Complex

The Problem

Burn injury to the anterior chest may produce:

a. Restriction of breast development by direct injury to breast tissue in the young female.

b. Distortion and loss of volume or contour in the older patient.

c. In either a or b, partial or complete destruction of the nipple-areola complex.

The injury may be confined to one breast or may affect both. Augmentation mammaplasty using silicone-gel prostheses may be indicated for re-creation of breast volume and contour when the healed burn has resulted in pliable scar. The prosthesis is usually placed beneath the remaining breast tissue and above the pectoralis muscle fascia. If the breast and soft tissue have been destroyed, resulting in a bed of scar, the implant should be placed beneath the pectoralis major muscle. Although there may be somewhat less projection of the breast with a submuscular prosthesis, a more vascular protective cover is provided that lessens the risk of implant extrusion. Various methods are available for reconstruction of the damaged or absent nipple-areola complex at a later operative procedure.

Technique

Figures 43–1, 43–2, 43–3. This patient (courtesy of William C. Trier, M.D.) has bilateral loss of breast volume caused by injury before puberty, distortion of the right nipple-areola structures, and nearly complete loss of the left nipple and areola. The overlying skin and remaining breast tissue were adequate for submammary placement of silicone-gel prostheses.

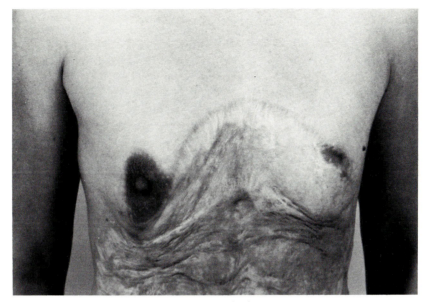
Figure 43-1

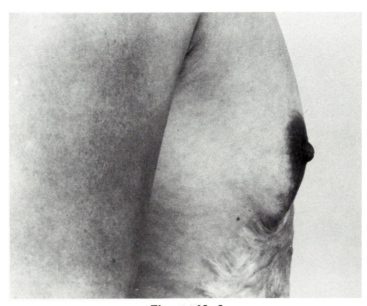
Figure 43-2

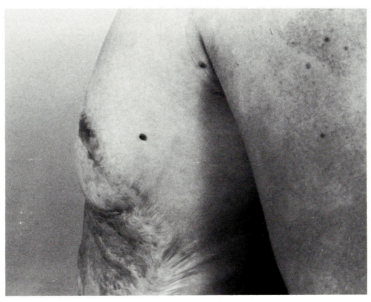
Figure 43-3

Figure 43-4. The inframammary folds were marked preoperatively, lying on a line from midhumerus to midhumerus, projected across the chest wall. The nipple-areola complex will ultimately lie approximately 5 to 6 cm superior to the inframammary fold. An incision 6 to 8 cm long is made, 1 cm above the inframammary fold, and located centrally. The incision is deepened to expose the pectoralis fascia. A submammary pocket, extending 1 to 2 cm from the midline superiorly to the infraclavicular fossa, laterally to the anterior axillary line, and inferiorly to the inframammary fold, is made with blunt dissection. Care is taken to remain above the pectoralis fascia, and any blood vessels encountered are coagulated with an electric cautery.

Lighted, fiberoptic retractors are useful in the procedure, as are headlights, so that direct vision in this submammary pocket is achieved.

The appropriate prosthesis was selected preoperatively (by the patient and surgeon), by having her wear a supportive bra and trying different implants to give an approximation of the size required for symmetry.

The prostheses are placed in the submammary pocket, and the incision is closed with synthetic 4-0 absorbable suture material in the subcutaneous tissue and dermis. A continuous 4-0 monofilament suture is used for intradermal closure of the skin. Small, adhesive strips are added to support the closure, and covered with a single layer of dry gauze dressing. A fitted surgical bra is placed on the patient, completing the dressing.

Postoperatively, gross arm movement is restricted for 10 days, at which time the skin suture is removed. The patient is given an additional bra so that a clean one is available, and these are worn day and night for three weeks.

Figure 43-5. If the overlying skin and remaining breast tissue are judged to be inadequate for submammary placement of a prosthesis, it is placed beneath the pectoralis major muscle. The initial incision is identical to the one used for submammary augmentation of the breast. However, as the incision is deepened, the fascia and border of the pectoralis muscle are identified laterally. The fascia is incised, and a plane of dissection is developed beneath the pectoralis major muscle. The medial insertions of this muscle to the lower ribs may be incised, allowing evaluation of the extent of the muscle. Bleeding points here must be carefully controlled under direct vision to avoid hematoma formation. The prosthesis is placed into the submuscular pocket, and the pectoralis muscle is draped over it. The previously incised fascia may be sutured inferiorly to maintain the breast prosthesis in position.

Figure 43-6. The patient in Figures 43-1 to 43-4 is seen several months after submammary augmentation mammaplasty. The right nipple-areola complex has become stretched and remodeled as a result of the underlying prosthesis. The right areola is actually larger than most patients desire, exceeding the usual 4- to 5-cm diameter that is normal for most individuals. Unfortunately, this patient would not permit an areola-sharing technique for reduction of the right areola and reconstruction of the left nipple-areola complex. Therefore, by measuring the distance from the midclavicular line and sternal notch to the nipple, a site over the left breast was chosen with respect to location and size to match the large right areola. The circular area is de-epithelialized in preparation for receiving a free graft for areolar reconstruction.

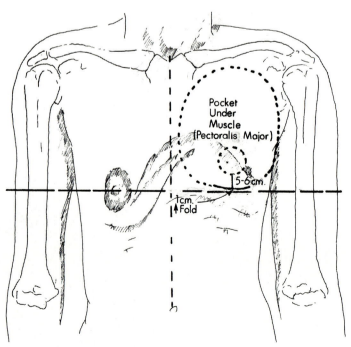

Figure 43-4

LOSS OF BREAST VOLUME AND DESTRUCTION OF THE NIPPLE-AREOLA COMPLEX

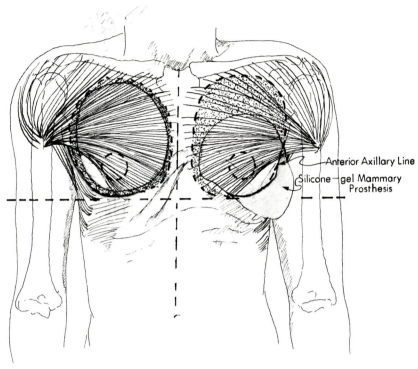

Figure 43-5

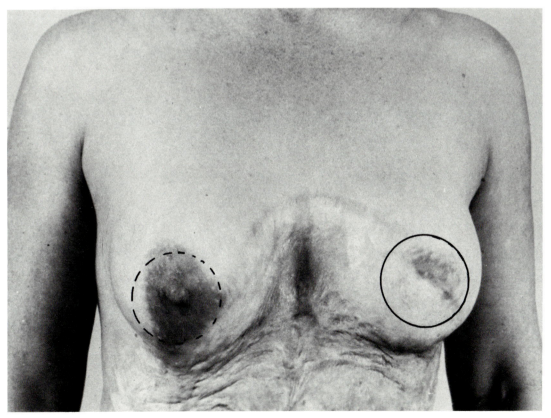

Figure 43-6

Figure 43-7. The labium minus was chosen for a graft. A semicircular, full-thickness excision of the margin of the labium minus is made, with the diameter equal to that of the areolar recipient site. The graft is then dissected so that it opens into a circular structure and is transferred to the recipient site upon the breast. Fine, interrupted sutures are used to maintain the position of the labial graft, and a light, nonadherent dressing is applied beneath a properly fitting bra for support.

Figures 43-8, 43-9, 43-10. The patient is shown six months after areolar reconstruction. Further stretching of the areola following augmentation has occurred, resulting in symmetrical but rather large areolae. The patient had further declined creation of a nipple for the left breast. A disadvantage of the labium minus graft is seen here: considerable contrast in pigmentation with respect to the normal areola on the left. This patient did achieve good breast contour and symmetry, but the result was not optimal because of the size and color of the areolae. This might have been obviated if she had accepted another reconstructive technique.

Pitfalls and Solutions

1. Preoperative planning for a correctly sized prosthesis is necessary to avoid asymmetry and patient dissatisfaction.

2. Preoperative marking of the inframammary folds and proposed sites for areolar reconstruction must be carried out. This will avoid errors made by marking the supine and anesthetized patient in the operating room.

3. The patient should acquire a full understanding of the available methods for reconstruction of the nipple-areola complex. Disadvantages of each procedure with respect to size, color, and texture must be outlined. If the patient cannot accept a particular technique, the reconstruction can be done only if she understands the possible failure of a technique that is less acceptable to the surgeon.

4. Hemostasis in either the submammary or subpectoral augmentation procedure is mandatory. Hematoma formation will require reoperation, and may cause further scarring and asymmetry.

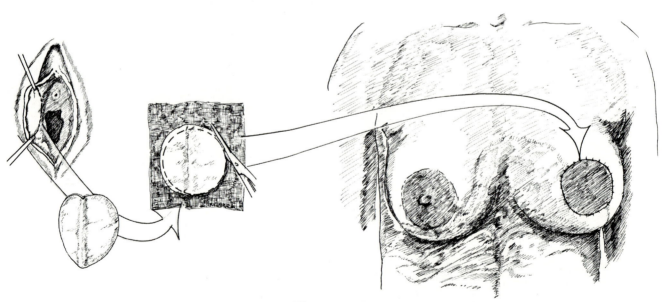

Figure 43-7

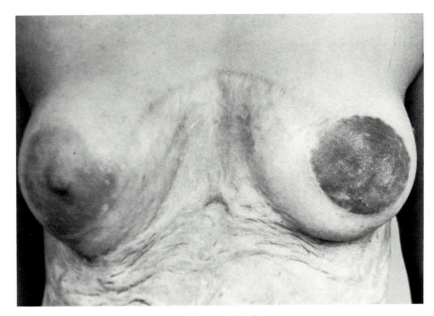

Figure 43-8

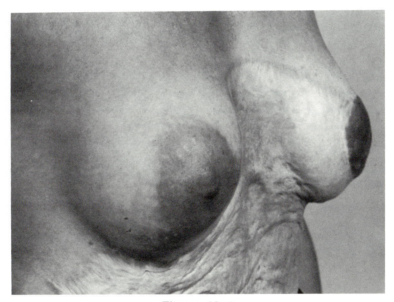

Figure 43-9

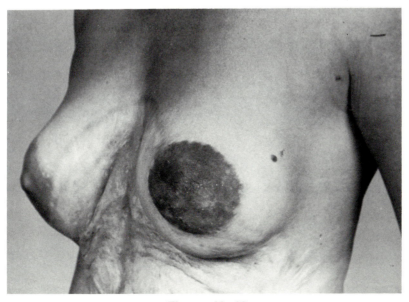

Figure 43-10

44

Reconstruction of the Nipple-Areola Complex

The Problem

The nipple-areola complex is often distorted or completely destroyed when the breast is burned. Once the volume and contour of the injured breast is restored, the patient usually desires reconstruction of the complex. As previously mentioned, it is best to delay reconstruction of the nipple and areolar structures until sometime after initial breast reconstructive surgery. If this is attempted at the primary reconstructive procedure, edema of the breast may lead to inadequate healing of the nipple and areolar tissues. Further, after breast augmentation procedures, the overlying breast skin will remodel and stretch with time, making location and estimation of size more difficult if done early. After several months, final contour of the reconstructed breast is apparent, and nipple-areola reconstruction carried out at this time will yield better esthetic results.

There are several different procedures for the creation of the areola and nipple. As indicated earlier, labium minus free grafts may be used when both areolae require restoration. However, the pigmentation of most labial grafts is more intense than the normal areola. Thus, in unilateral reconstruction, another method is suggested in order to obtain a closer color match.

Technique

Figure 44–1. This patient previously had release of scar contractures of the right breast, and reduction of the size of both breasts to achieve better volume symmetry. Skin markings indicate the proposed location of the new areolae, in the midclavicular line, and with their inferior margins approximately 6 cm superior to the inframammary fold.

Figure 44–2. The upper inner thigh is a suitable donor site. Skin in this area is hairless, and has a slightly darker pigmentation than the usual skin of the breasts. The pigmentation is less, however, than that of the labia minora.

A full-thickness, rectangular skin graft is excised from the upper inner thigh, measuring approximately 4 to 5 by 8 to 10 cm, and transferred to a moist gauze. The donor site is closed directly by excision of a triangular segment of skin from each end of the rectangle, and approximation of the skin edges with inverted, synthetic, absorbable sutures and a running, 4-0 monofilament, nonabsorbable suture.

The circular recipient sites on each breast are de-epithelialized. Circular areolar grafts with a diameter of 4 to 5 cm are then cut from the rectangular, full-thickness graft. These are sutured into the recipient sites on the breasts with 5-0 monofilament suture. A nonadherent dressing is applied, and a well fitting bra placed over this in the operating room. The bra and dressing are maintained in place continuously, with one or two inspections of the grafts during the first ten postoperative days. Sutures are removed on the tenth day after surgery.

Figure 44–3. The patient is shown a few weeks after surgery. She did not want reconstruction of the nipple itself, which could have been done during the initial recreation of the areolae.

Nipple sharing is a useful method when one normal nipple-areola complex is present. This may be done as either: (a) full-thickness sharing, using a portion of the normal areola and nipple; or (b) split-thickness sharing, using a thin section of the entire area of a normal areola and nipple.

RECONSTRUCTION OF THE NIPPLE-AREOLA COMPLEX

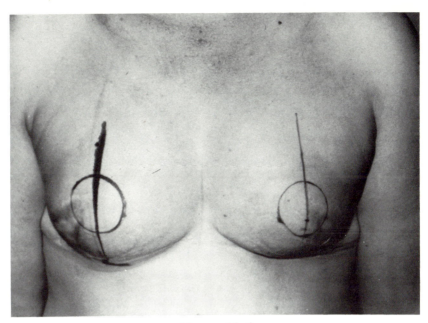

Figure 44–1

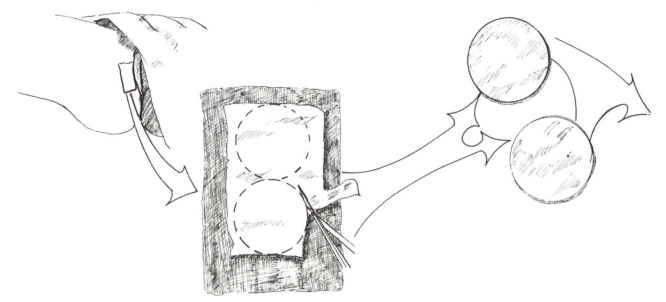

Figure 44–2

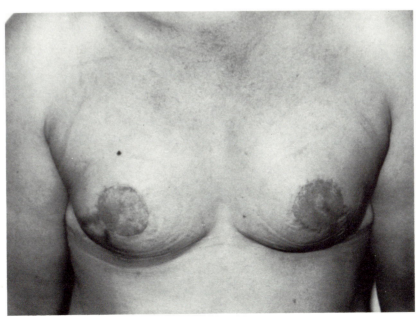

Figure 44–3

Figure 44-4. The full-thickness method is appropriate when the intact nipple-areola complex is larger than the usual 4 to 5 cm in diameter. The shaded area is excised at the level of the subcutaneous tissue, and retained. The resulting upper semicircular portion of the normal nipple-areola complex is incised at its margin, and undermined for a few millimeters above its diameter. The skin edges surrounding the undermined structure are advanced, and the undermined areola is drawn inferiorly and sutured in the midline. The margins are then sutured to the surrounding breast skin edges with interrupted 5-0 monofilament sutures. This reduces the size of the initial areola by one-third to one-half.

The excised semicircular portion is then transferred to the other breast, where a recipient site is prepared by de-epithelializing a circular area with a diameter of 4 to 5 cm. The graft is then sutured at the margins superiorly, and the lower portion approximated in the midline inferiorly, as was the donor area.

When there is one intact nipple-areola complex of reasonable size, or when a patient desires matching of the intact structure regardless of its area, a split-thickness method of nipple-areola sharing is useful.

Figure 44-5. This method of reconstruction is illustrated. A recipient site is de-epithelialized, and its area and location matched with the intact nipple-areola complex of the ipsilateral breast. Using a drum dermatome with adhesive dermatome tape in place, an area equivalent to that of the intact nipple-areola structure is removed from the dermatome tape, exposing only the base adhesive for this area. With the dermatome set to take a split-thickness graft 0.012 inches in thickness, the dermatome is placed exactly over the donor nipple-areola. Pressure downward causes the nipple to be depressed slightly, and as the dermatome knife is manipulated in removing the graft, two separate segments will be removed as shown: the outer, doughnut-shaped areola portion; and a central, circular nipple portion. The areola portion is transferred to the recipient site after removal from the dermatome adhesive tape, and sutured into position with multiple 5-0 monofilament sutures. The central nipple portion is then sutured after a few buried, synthetic, absorbable sutures have been employed to compress and elevate the subcutaneous tissue in this central area. This will cause an elevation of the subcutaneous tissue over which the nipple graft is placed, giving projection to this structure. Nonadherent dressings and a supportive bra worn for seven days complete the procedure.

When only a nipple reconstruction is required, several methods may be considered. Free grafts using the plantar pad of the third or fourth toe have been used. Local procedures that involve undermining and suture of the subareolar tissues to create projection, with subsequent skin grafting, are possible.

Figure 44-6. A method is illustrated that employs the excision of several triangles of areolar epithelium surrounding a circular area 4 to 6 mm in diameter. The resultant defects are sutured side-to-side, creating projection and condensation of the surface, and yielding a contour and texture quite like a normal nipple.

Figure 44-7. Another method for producing definite projection and definition of the nipple is shown. A semicircular incision in the center of the normal areola is made, approximately 6 to 7 mm in diameter. Two trap door-shaped, rounded incisions are made in the postauricular skin, through which buttons of cartilage are harvested, 5 to 6 mm in diameter. The postauricular wounds are sutured, and the buttons stacked one on the other and placed in a small pocket dissected beneath the semicircular incision in the recipient areola. The wound is closed with interrupted sutures, and a light, protective dressing is placed beneath a well fitting bra.

Pitfalls and Solutions

1. For each of these procedures, careful patient education is required. Often the use of distant and seemingly unusual tissues for nipple-areola reconstruction may be difficult for a patient to understand and accept.

2. Although most of the nipple-areola reconstructive procedures can be carried out at the time of primary breast surgery, the result may be unpredictable. When final breast size and contour is achieved, identification of landmarks is facilitated, location and size of the new nipple-areola are easier to determine, and the ultimate result is usually better.

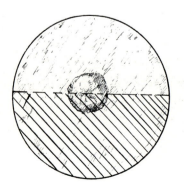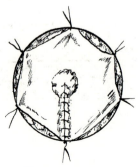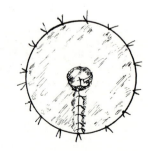

Figure 44-4

RECONSTRUCTION OF THE NIPPLE-AREOLA COMPLEX

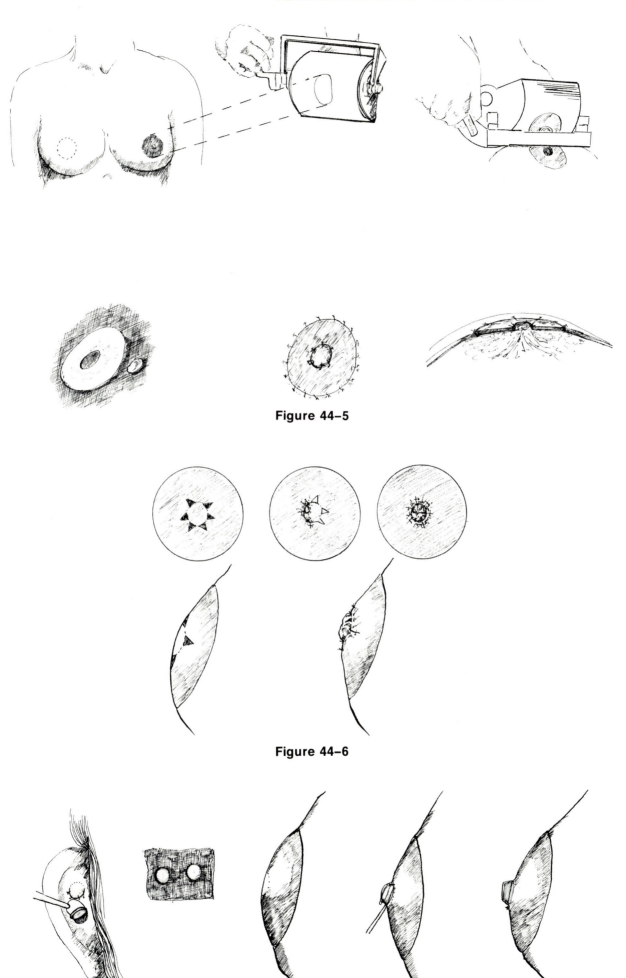

Figure 44-5

Figure 44-6

Figure 44-7

45

Breast Reconstruction Using the Latissimus Dorsi Myocutaneous Flap

The Problem

When deep truncal burns occur in the young female, deformities occur that may include:

a. Absent nipples and areolae.
b. Failure of normal breast development.
c. Severe, deep scarring to the level of the chest wall.
d. Any combination of these findings.

Figure 45–1. A female patient's anterior chest is shown several years following deep thermal injury (courtesy of J. Barry Bishop, M.D.). Multiple split-thickness skin grafts accomplished earlier resulted in healed wounds. Breast development at and after puberty was sparse because of intrinsic breast tissue injury. Constricting scar over the area worsened the situation. Small, silicone breast prostheses had actually been inserted beneath the healed wounds, but resulted in ill-defined, poorly contoured mounds with no nipple-areola structures. The patient desired further reconstruction.

Technique

Latissimus dorsi myocutaneous flaps were selected for resurfacing the anterior chest wall, with appropriately sized breast prostheses placed beneath the flaps in a single operative procedure. The nipple-areola complex would be reconstructed in a second procedure. In this patient the posterior chest was unburned, but in other patients the identical type of flap has been raised safely and transposed even when the area had been skin-grafted. Intimate knowledge of the anatomy of the latissimus dorsi muscle, its fascia, vascular supply, and surrounding landmarks is required. Cadaver dissection is imperative in order to gain sufficient experience to perform this procedure safely.

Figure 45–2. The anterior two-thirds to three-quarters of the latissimus dorsi muscle is supplied by the thoracodorsal artery and vein, branches of the axillary artery and vein respectively. Perforating vessels course upward from the deep surface of the muscle and enter the overlying skin, providing circulation so that the myocutaneous latissimus dorsi flap is predictable and reliable. (The details of the anatomy and surgical dissection have been elucidated by McGraw, Bostwick, Nahai, Wallace, and Vasconez.)

BREAST RECONSTRUCTION USING THE LATISSIMUS DORSI MYOCUTANEOUS FLAP

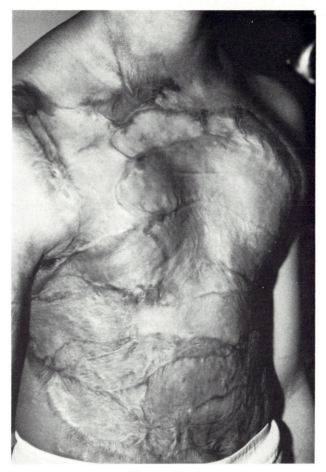

Figure 45-1

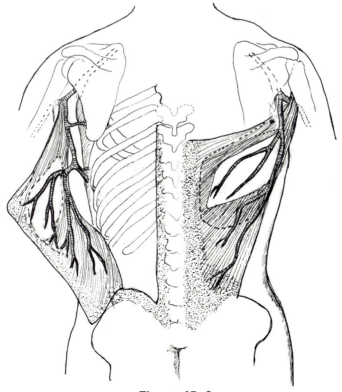

Figure 45-2

Figure 45–3. Preoperatively the anterior and posterior chest walls are examined, and markings for the donor flap and recipient site are made. The skin incision over the back for each flap is marked roughly in the center of the expanse of the latissimus dorsi muscle beneath, using the scapula, vertebral column, posterior iliac crest, and posterior margin of the axilla as boundaries. The resulting skin markings for the cutaneous portion of the flap will generally measure 8 to 10 cm in width by 20 to 25 cm in length, describing an ovoid- to diamond-shaped area. Anteriorly the inframammary fold is marked at a point on the anterior chest wall equivalent to the level of the midhumerus. This will also mark the inferior position of the chest excision wound. A similar area with an ovoid- to diamond-shape is then marked on the anterior chest, centering the area over a point where the final nipple-areola complex will be situated. This point will be approximately 5 cm superior to the inframammary fold, and 1 to 2 cm lateral to the midclavicular line. When the incisional markings are completed, the patient and surgeon choose the proper size for the breast prostheses. A soft, easily adjusted bra is used, and various-sized implants are placed within the bra so that the patient can estimate the resulting contour. The bra should have a reasonably wide back band so that the patient can appreciate the fact that the final closure of the donor site will largely be hidden beneath the bra posteriorly. Generally, a breast prosthesis no larger than 250 cc should be chosen for a patient of average height and weight. Too large a prosthesis may result in compromise of the vascular supply to the flap from internal pressure.

The patient is placed prone on the operating table, and the entire posterior chest down to the gluteal areas is prepared. The initial incision is made approximately 3 to 4 cm in front of the anterior border of the latissimus dorsi muscle. This border is easily palpable when the subcutaneous tissue is exposed through an initial 8- to 10-cm incision along the preoperative markings. The latissimus dorsi is then elevated from the underlying serratus anterior. This step is most important, since entry into the incorrect fascial plane will result in inability to elevate the flap correctly when the final incisions are completed. The entire latissimus dorsi muscle can be undermined by blunt dissection from this wound. At a point approximately 10 to 12 cm below the apex of the axillary fossa, the vascular pedicle to this flap can be palpated and then visualized by continuing the dissection anteriorly and superiorly. The previously marked skin incision is completed, outlining the cutaneous portion of the flap. The depth of the incision is only to the fascia overlying the latissimus dorsi muscle. After completing this incision, the periphery is undermined *away* from the cutaneous flap, and deepened down toward the scapula, vertebral column, and posterior iliac crest to expose the extent of the muscle and its fascial insertions. This fascia is incised, 3 to 5 cm from the superior border of the previously marked skin island, which is 8 to 10 cm lateral to the vertebral column, and 6 to 10 cm superior to the posterior iliac crest. These incisions will then connect the spaces previously created by undermining the latissimus dorsi muscle, and will overlie the serratus anterior muscle. The flap must be elevated from the periphery toward the vascular pedicle, in order to keep the central skin island applied to the muscle and avoid avulsing it during operative maneuvers.

Figure 45–4. The entire myocutaneous flap is then elevated, with any necessary dissection in the region of the vascular pedicle being carried out under direct vision. A branch of the thoracodorsal artery to the serratus anterior muscle may be divided if any additional arc of rotation is required. The thoracodorsal artery to the myocutaneous flap must not be injured. The posterior incision is now closed, using 4-0 synthetic, absorbable material in the dermis, and 4-0 monofilament sutures in the skin. A suction catheter is placed in each of the posterior wounds and brought out below the operative incisions.

The patient is then lifted in the prone position, and carefully supinated with the arms extended so that the flap can be held anteriorly as the anterior chest is prepared and draped for surgery.

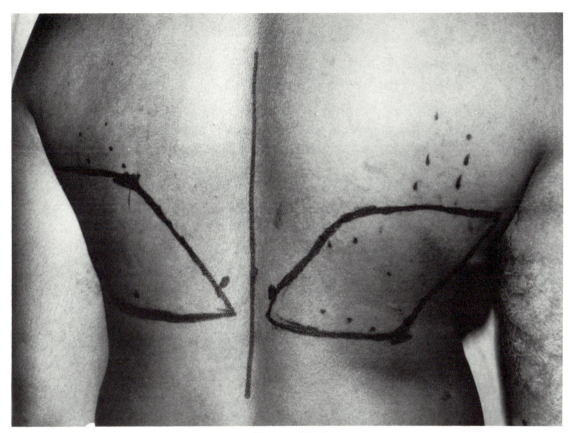

Figure 45-3

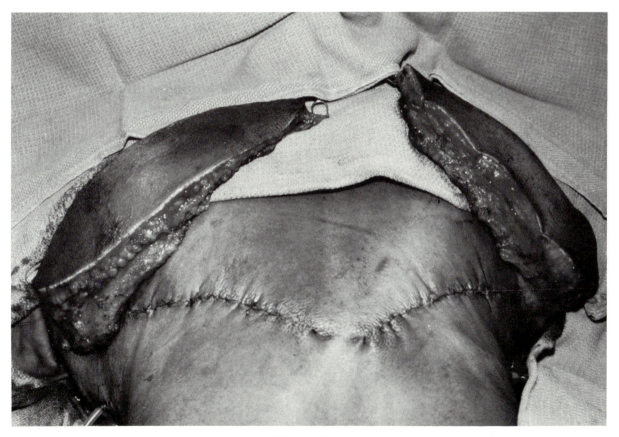

Figure 45-4

Figure 45-5. An incision from the anterior margin of the donor wound is carried below the axillary fold to connect with the anterior chest wall markings. This provides a site for the vascular pedicle when the flap is inset.

The anterior incisions are made, excising the burn scar within the perimeter of the markings to whatever depth it extends to. The previously chosen prostheses are placed in position in the center of the resulting defect, and the myocutaneous flap is draped over the prostheses. The muscular extensions of the flap are adjusted, and if undermining at the periphery of the excised recipient site is required for placement of the muscle, it is done at this time. The muscle is then fixed at its peripheral margins to the chest wall with absorbable sutures. With the prostheses covered by muscle, the skin of the chest is approximated to the skin of the flap with synthetic, absorbable, subcuticular sutures and interrupted, monofilament skin sutures. Suction catheters are placed in the wound, and brought out laterally and below the chest incisions. Only loose, nonadherent dressings are applied to the wounds, so that no additional pressure is added to the flaps that could compromise their vascular supply.

Figure 45-6. Approximately four months later the patient had a secondary nipple-areola reconstruction on the newly created breast mounds. Upper, inner thigh, full-thickness skin grafts were used for the areolae, and volar, toe-pad, free grafts for the nipples, as described by Bishop and Bostwick.

Pitfalls and Solutions

1. Careful markings of the incisions and selection of the proper breast prostheses must be accomplished preoperatively. These decisions cannot be made on the operating table.

2. The anterior portion of the incision to expose the border of the latissimus dorsi muscle should be made first. The serratus anterior muscle provides a landmark to prevent entry into the incorrect fascial plane.

3. Through the anterior incision, dissection and visualization of the vascular pedicle is accomplished, avoiding injury to this structure.

4. The flap should be elevated from the periphery at the musculofascial level, toward the vascular pedicle, preventing undue manipulation that might cause avulsion of the skin from the underlying latissimus dorsi muscle.

5. Drainage, together with supportive but nonconstricting dressings, is essential in the postoperative period.

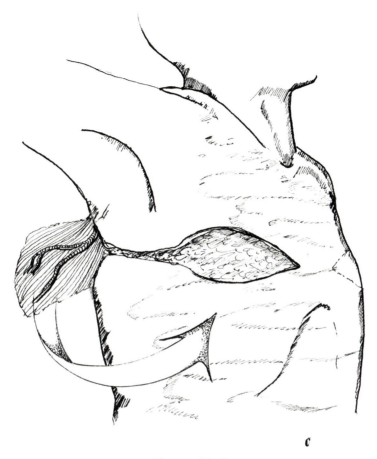

Figure 45-5

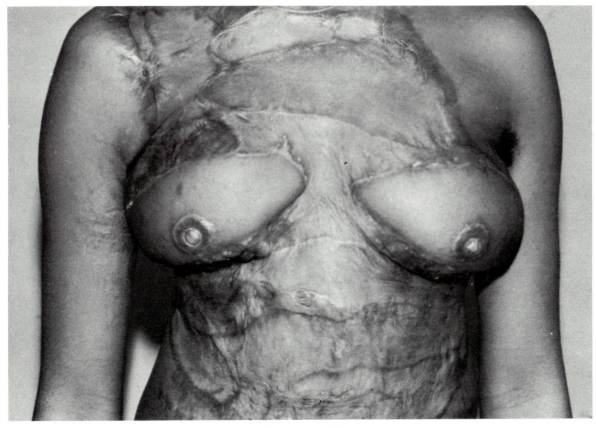

Figure 45-6

46

Burns of the Genitalia

The Problem

Burns of the female genitalia are rare because the structures are well protected. Burns of the male genitalia are more common and are often seen in conjunction with involvement of the lower abdomen, perineum, and inner thighs. Most common late presentations include:

a. Contracture with shortening and fixation to the lower abdomen, secondary to burns of the dorsum of the penile shaft and pubic area.

b. Webbing in the perineum and/or scrotum.

c. Hypospadias secondary to deep burns of the volar penis and scrotum.

d. Total dysfunction of the penis and/or scrotum secondary to deep burns.

Technique

Figure 46–1A, B. A combination of these problems is demonstrated. Anterior and posterior webbing exists, and the penis is not grossly present or palpable. If it exists, it is pulled superiorly by wound contracture.

Figure 46–2. Testicles are not palpable, and the patient is able to void only when sitting.

Figure 46–3. This situation obviously cannot be reconstructed in one operation, so that the first effort is an exploratory one to determine what normal anatomy remains. The pubis is marked with an "x" as an anterior landmark above the genitalia, and the anus is marked posteriorly. Incisions are drawn along the contractile webs of the perineum. Superior to the inguinal ligament they will converge toward the pubis.

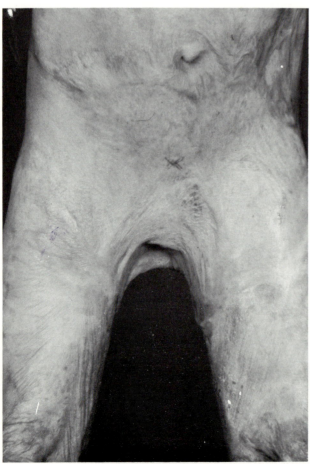

Figure 46–1A

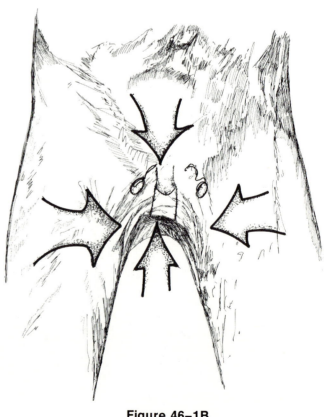

Figure 46–1B

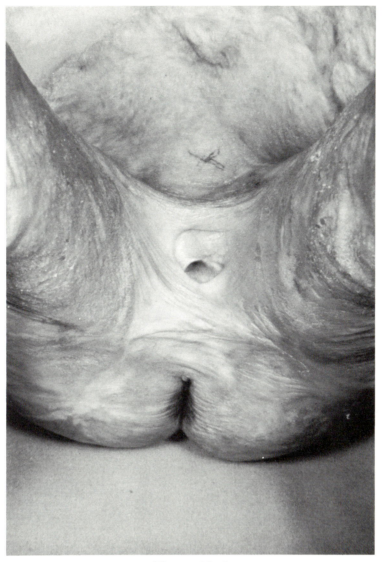

Figure 46-2

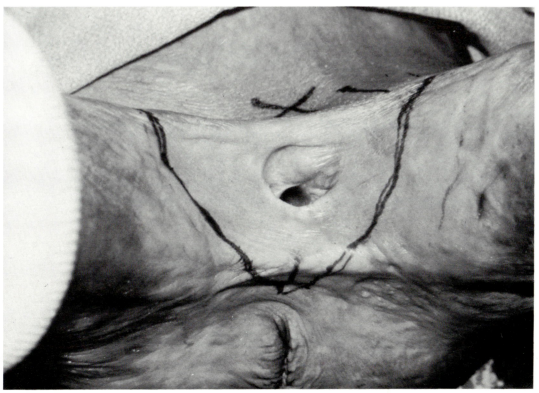

Figure 46-3

Figure 46-4. A urinary catheter must be inserted initially, to give some indication of the position of the urethra and of what remains of the penile shaft. Incision and dissection are begun on the superior thigh so that, if the testicles are present, they can be protected by a central mass of tissue. As the released tissue is retracted superiorly, a large thigh defect becomes apparent, a contracted penis is palpable, and the testicles are visualized. The vascular pedicles are identified to avoid damage, dissected, and sutured caudally as far as the shortened cord and vas allow. Because it is impossible to make the testicles descend to a normal position, it is obvious that a further procedure will be needed; thus, the position of the testicles is marked with several blue monofilament sutures. They are then covered by the central mass of tissue, and split-thickness skin grafts are applied to the thighs. The release achieved at stage 1 allows for: (a) extracorporeal placement of the testicles; and (b) identification of a mound of tissue (penis) in which the urethra is located.

All defects are grafted in the anticipation that some recurrence of contracture will occur. It is an axiom of burn reconstruction to overcorrect a contracture release and splint the operative site for nine to 12 months. Obviously it is impossible to splint this wound satisfactorily, and some contracture of the grafted wound must be expected.

Figure 46-5. At stage 2, six months later, a mound (penis) is present, the testicles are palpable in a somewhat superior location (*x*), and the contractures are less severe.

Figure 46-6. Incision of the thighs bilaterally allows a lateral-to-medial dissection.

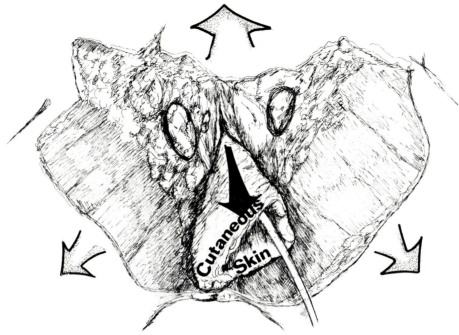

Figure 46-4

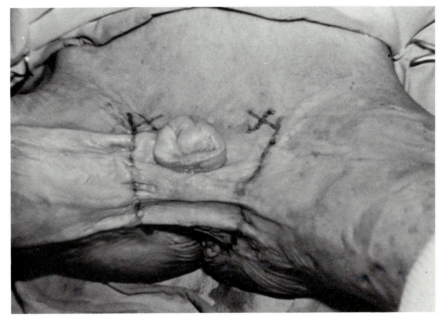

Figure 46-5

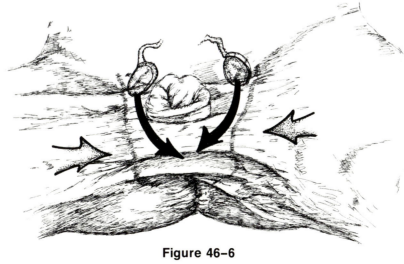

Figure 46-6

TRUNK, GENITALIA, AND LOWER EXTREMITY

Figure 46–7A, B. Identification of the testicles is simplified by sutures that had been left to mark their location (identified by the forceps). Total mobilization is now possible without devascularizing the testicles, and they are placed under the pseudoscrotum (the central tissue).

Figure 46–8A, B. The central tissue is sutured down around the testicles, creating the pseudoscrotum. The thigh wounds are covered with split-thickness skin grafts, and the legs splinted in abduction for ten days. A "beehive" dressing is placed around the penis, and the urinary catheter held on mild tension to keep the shaft elevated, to reduce edema. The patient is then allowed out of the splint during the day, with sponge rubber conformers placed over the grafts to maintain abduction of the thighs. The splint is worn at night for six months.

Figure 46–9. Two years later the appearance is much improved and the patient voids normally. Definitive penis resurfacing, if required, will be done when the child is older, as continued emphasis on this problem might affect him even more psychologically.

Recurrent webbing of the perineum may be managed by Z-plasties, or additional skin replacement in the future.

Pitfalls and Solutions

1. Distortion of the anatomy in perineal burns is the rule, and inadvertent amputation of the penis or devascularization of the testes can occur during exploration and contracture release.

2. Insert a catheter before surgery so that the course of the penis can be easily traced.

3. Dissect laterally to medially, from a recognizable, safe anatomical landmark such as the thigh to the unknown, whether it be scrotum, penile shaft, or urethra.

4. Make sure the patient and family understand that these are staged procedures. The surgeon must avoid the temptation of trying to correct everything at once.

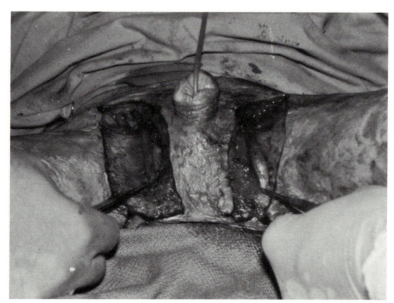

Figure 46–7A

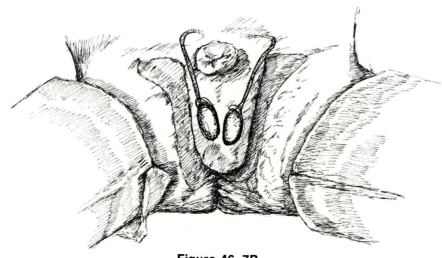

Figure 46–7B

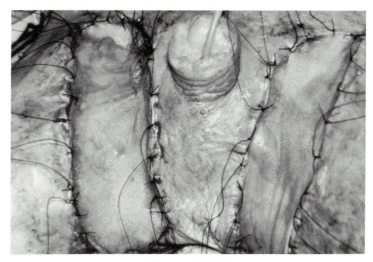

Figure 46-8A

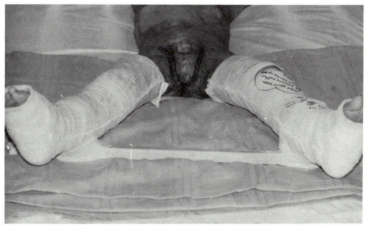

Figure 46-8B

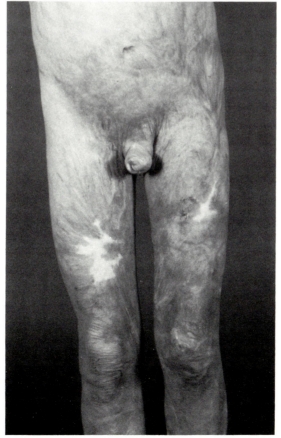

Figure 46-9

47

Reconstruction of the Groin: The Tensor Fasciae Latae Myocutaneous Flap

The Problem

Isolated burn injuries of the groins are uncommon in thermal trauma, but can occur quite frequently as a result of irradiation injury. Hypertrophic scarring across the groin from abdomen to perineum or thigh in large thermal burns usually can be managed by excision and split-thickness skin grafting. However, in the irradiation injury, there may be scarring, decreased vascular supply, and compromise of the integrity of a large area of skin and subcutaneous tissue. Major vascular channels may be exposed following excision of these deep and extensive wounds. Well vascularized, durable, and sizeable amounts of composite tissue are required to resurface such defects.

Mathes and Nahai have demonstrated the safety and versatility of the tensor fasciae latae myocutaneous flap. This flap may be used for a wide variety of resurfacing problems over the trochanters, groins, and perineum, and posteriorly over the sacrum. Clinically the tensor fasciae latae myocutaneous flap is predictable, has a remarkable area of useful skin compared with the small size of the included muscle, and does not sacrifice significant muscular functional loss when translocated.

Figure 47-1. The tensor fasciae latae muscle originates on the anterior outer rim of the iliac crest, and inserts into the iliotibial tract of the lateral thigh. Its arterial supply comes from the lateral circumflex branch of the profunda femoris artery as a single, dominant pedicle. Significantly, this vessel enters the deep surface of the tensor fasciae latae muscle, traverses it, and sends numerous musculocutaneous perforators to a large area of skin overlying the small muscle, and distally to the skin of the lateral thigh, to within 6 cm of the knee. Therefore, the muscle may be elevated on its dominant pedicle, which enters it 8 to 10 cm below the anterior superior iliac spine, with varying lengths of overlying skin extending well beyond the muscle itself. The width of the skin may be from 6 to 15 cm.

Figure 47-2. A patient is shown on the operating table, with markings indicating the location of the tensor fasciae latae muscle (cross-hatched area), the central width of the flap (15 cm in this patient), and the distal extent of this myocutaneous flap. The proximal, dominant arterial pedicle for the entire flap enters 8 to 10 cm below the anterior superior iliac spine, near the center of the cross-hatched area.

Figure 47-3. This illustration indicates the entry of the proximal pedicle, the lateral circumflex artery, and its distal ramifications nourishing the large area of skin of the anterolateral thigh. The arc of rotation, in this instance toward the groin, is shown. In other applications of this flap, the proximal skin overlying the muscle may be incised and the flap elevated as an island, allowing full 180-degree rotation superiorly to cover abdominal wall defects.

The anterior border of the tensor fasciae latae myocutaneous flap lies on a line made from the anterior superior iliac spine to the lateral condyle of the tibia. The posterior trochanter defines the width maximally, usually up to 15 cm.

This flap is elevated from its distal extent after the length required is determined. For simple groin coverage, approximately 30 cm of length are required, measured from the proximal arterial pedicle. The distal incision is made to expose the fascia lata, which is elevated with the overlying skin. As proximal dissection is begun, the skin margins are sutured to this fascia to prevent avulsion of the perforating vessels. The vastus lateralis muscle is exposed as the flap is elevated proximally. Dissection continues proximally until the region of the vascular pedicle is reached. It is not necessary to fully expose and skeletonize this pedicle for local rotation of the flap toward the groin. The tensor fasciae latae muscle is elevated with the flap, which is frequently rotated toward the groin, and tested to determine adequacy of length for the defect in question. Careful adherence to the landmarks, and performing the dissection from distal to proximal in the plane indicated, renders it unnecessary to evaluate the vascularity of this flap by the use of intravenous fluorescein, as is the case with certain other myocutaneous flaps.

RECONSTRUCTION OF THE GROIN: THE TENSOR FASCIAE LATAE MYOCUTANEOUS FLAP

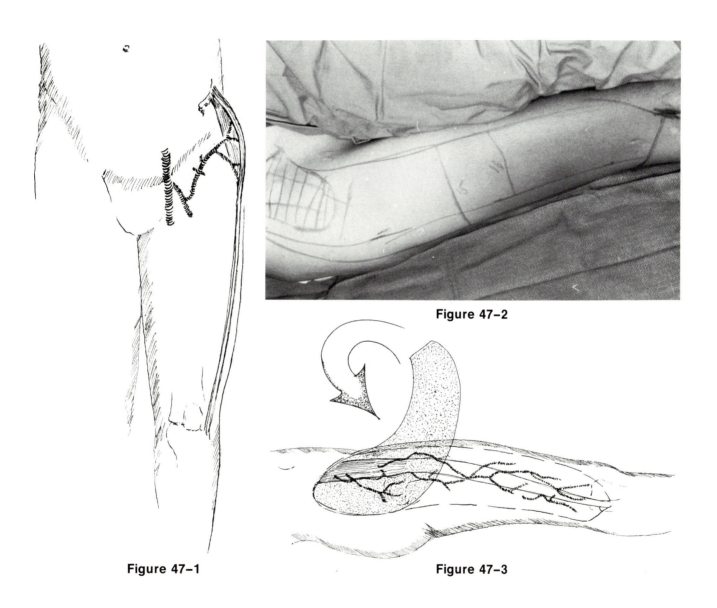

Figure 47-1

Figure 47-2

Figure 47-3

Figure 47-4. A patient is illustrated in whom scarring, unstable ulceration, and pain resulted following irradiation of the right groin several years previously for a localized, but metastatic, gynecological neoplasm. An area of groin skin measuring 27 by 12 cm was excised, including the damaged subcutaneous tissue, exposing the femoral vessels and deep musculature. In this patient a relatively short myocutaneous flap could be constructed. If the defect had extended medially, including the vulva, into the perineum, the flap would have been taken distally as needed to a limit within 6 cm of the knee. The flap has been elevated in the manner described and is lying *in situ*.

Figure 47-5. Anteriorly, the operative groin defect is fully visualized. Laterally, the skin of the myocutaneous flap has been sutured to the fascia lata to prevent injury to the perforating vessels during the course of the dissection.

Figure 47-6. The medial proximal portion of the myocutaneous flap has been incised to facilitate rotation toward the groin defect. In this way, buckling of the superior margin of the flap, which would cause a "dog-ear" near the anterior superior iliac spine, can be avoided. The translocated flap lies in position without tension.

Figure 47-7. The tensor fasciae latae myocutaneous flap is sutured into position with several 5-0 synthetic monofilament sutures. In about one-half of the patients, particularly those who are relatively obese, the lateral thigh donor defect may be closed primarily, without skin grafting. The patient illustrated required a small graft laterally at the upper margin of the thigh wound. Bed rest is maintained for three days, followed by supervised ambulation with elastic stockings in place.

Pitfalls and Solutions

1. Preoperative skin marking and palpation of landmarks are essential. Patients must be informed that skin grafting may be required to close all or part of the lateral thigh defect.

2. Strict adherence to the anatomical landmarks, using distal-to-proximal dissection, and protection of the proximal vascular pedicle will yield a safe, generous, and predictable flap for resurfacing defects of the groin and nearby areas.

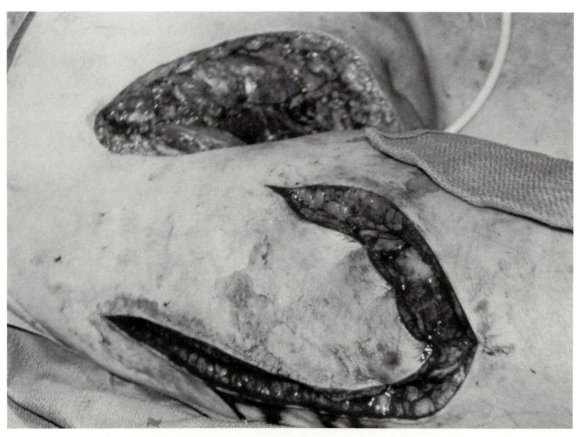

Figure 47-4

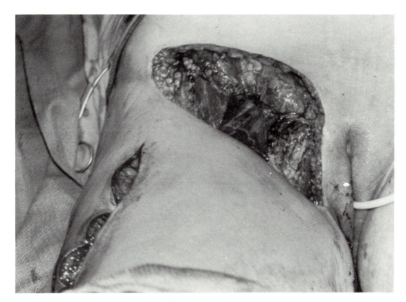

Figure 47–5

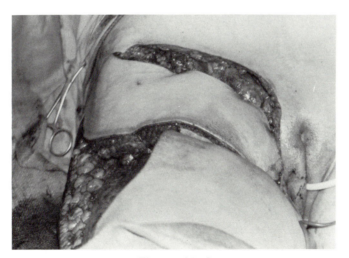

Figure 47–6

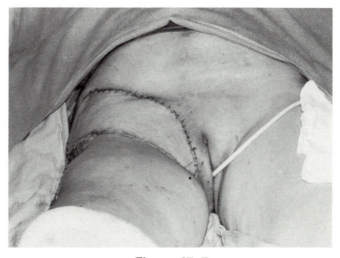

Figure 47–7

48

Contractures of the Knee

The Problem

The knee is often involved with contractures resulting from lateral or posterolateral burn scar. In contradistinction to the region of the elbow, however, local skin flaps are not usually adequate for relief of such contractures. The arrangement of the posterior thigh musculature, with insertions distal to the knee joint on either side, create a much deeper fossa in comparison with the elbow. At the elbow the insertions of the biceps and brachialis muscles create a more central, shallower fossa. In the event of a significant burn scar contracture of the popliteal fossa, hamstring muscle release and skin graft coverage may be required, since there is inadequate lateral tissue (as is often present at the elbow) for local pedicle coverage.

Technique

Figure 48–1. This medial knee contracture in a teenager is rather superficial, but restricts full extension of the knee and prevents his participation in sports. A small, chronic ulcer occurring in unstable, peripatellar, healed burned skin is also present and is of concern because of the possibility of future malignant degeneration.

Figure 48–2. The planned incision for a simple Z-plasty utilizes supple local skin that was present in this patient. The unstable dorsal scar is outlined for excision and split-thickness skin grafting.

Figures 48–3, 48–4. The development of the two Z-plasty flaps is done by wide local undermining in the subcutaneous plane, just above the muscular fascia. Small perforating vessels are carefully coagulated or ligated with absorbable suture material. The proposed transposition Z-plasty flaps will change the direction of tension from one parallel to the axis of the leg to a direction parallel to the axis of flexion and extension of the knee. The flaps are made sufficiently large to achieve closure of the wound under no tension when the knee is in full extension. The limbs of the Z-plasty flaps must equal the length of the incision/excision of the original linear scar contracture, and are incised at an angle of from 45 to 60 degrees. Care is taken not to undercut or thin the tips of the flaps. They are elevated, and held with skin hooks to further avoid compromising their vascularity.

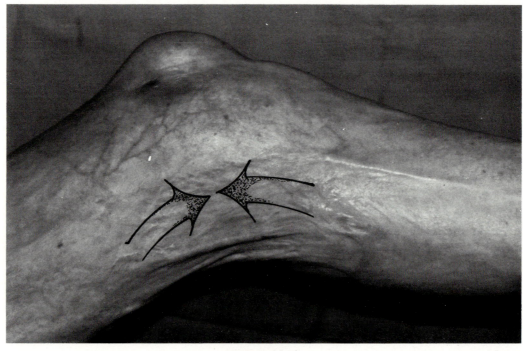

Figure 48–1

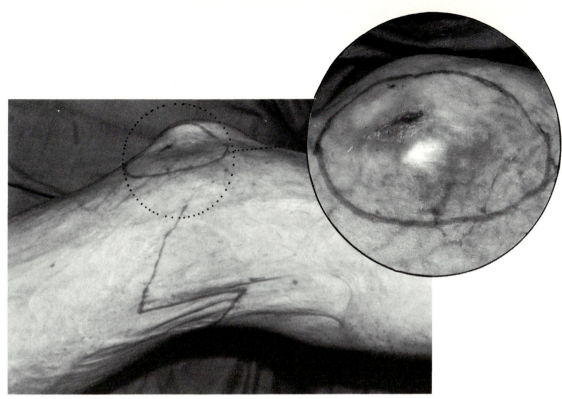

Figure 48–2

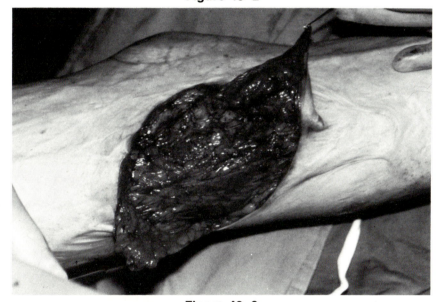

Figure 48–3

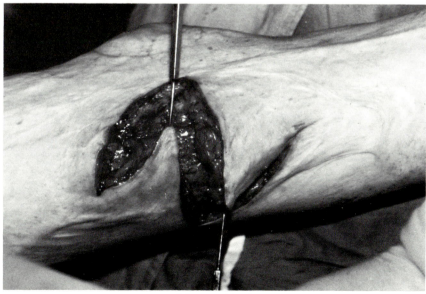

Figure 48–4

Figure 48–5. The flaps are sutured in their new position without tension. Interrupted, inverted sutures of 4–0 synthetic, absorbable material are used in the subcuticular layer to position the transposed flaps. Continuous, subcuticular, 5–0 monofilament, nonabsorbable suture is used for final skin approximation. This suture is left in place for three weeks to assure satisfactory healing. The leg is maintained for ten days, postoperatively with 30 degrees of flexion of the knee by means of a posterior splint, to avoid tension on the healing wound. This is followed by gradual flexion and extension exercises, and weight-bearing.

Figure 48–6. Three months postoperatively the patient has full extension of the previously contracted knee, and a healed skin graft.

Pitfalls and Solutions

1. The Z-plasty flaps must be marked and constructed with sufficient size so that coverage is achieved with the knee in full extension, or residual limitation of motion will result.

2. Undermining and release of the skin flaps from their subcutaneous attachments must be adequate to allow them to be sutured without tension in the transposed location.

3. Postoperative splinting and immobilization of the leg with 30 degrees of flexion at the knee must be maintained for ten days, or until the flaps are healed adequately. If unrestricted motion occurs before this time, dehiscence of the wounds or hematoma, leading to flap necrosis, may result.

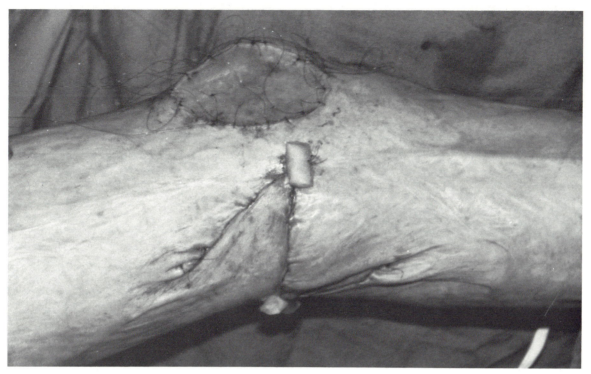

Figure 48–5

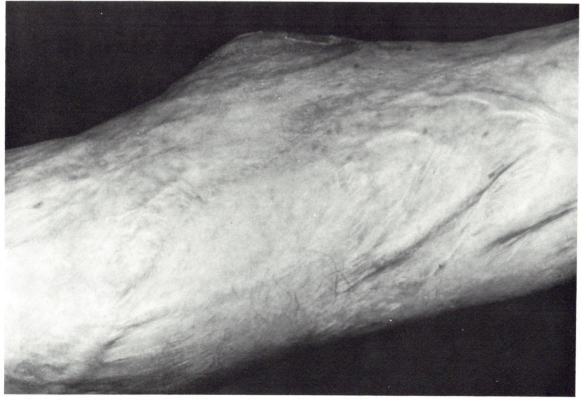

Figure 48–6

49

Knee: The Lateral Gastrocnemius Myocutaneous Flap

The Problem

Burn defects over the anterolateral aspect of the knee and upper tibia require durable and dependable coverage. Chronic wounds in these areas are notoriously unstable, causing disability and recurrent ulceration from local trauma. Over many years, the possibility of the development of Marjolin's ulcer carcinoma in these chronic wounds is prominent. The lateral gastrocnemius myocutaneous flap, as described by McGraw, is useful for these defects.

Figures 49–1, 49–2. A chronically ulcerated wound over the lateral aspect of the knee, with exposure of the joint space, is shown.

Technique

Both lower extremities are prepared and draped in the sterile field, to allow access for dissection and the acquisition of donor skin grafts from the upper thighs and buttock areas.

Figure 49–3. The vascular supply of the lateral head of the gastrocnemius muscle is very constant, and enters the proximal portion of the deep surface of the muscle 1 or 2 cm distal to the popliteal crease. Direct arterial branches from the popliteal artery enter the deep surface of the muscle after coursing for from 3 to 5 cm through the soft tissues near the popliteal crease. Accompanying veins drain into the popliteal vein. The sural nerve supplies lateral branches that innervate the muscle. Vessels pass through the muscle, and anastomose in the subdermal and dermal plexuses of the skin overlying the entire extent of this muscle. The lateral head of the gastrocnemius muscle ends distally at the midcalf.

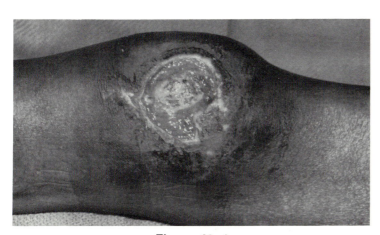

Figure 49-1

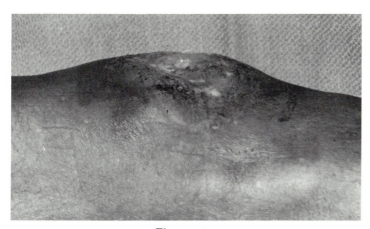

Figure 49-2

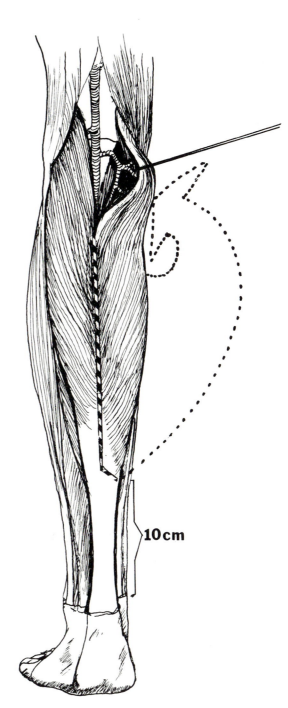

Figure 49-3

Figure 49-4. Incisions are planned so that the anterior margin of the flap will lie at the anterior border of the fibula, and the posterior margin of the flap will be at the posterior midline of the calf. A tourniquet may be used safely to simplify the dissection in a bloodless field. The proximal parts of the incisions are made just distal to the head of the fibula, distal to the popliteal crease. This portion of the incision is made first, progressing deep in the subcutaneous tissue to expose the juncture of the lateral and medial heads of the gastrocnemius muscle. At this level, the fascia is exposed and incised longitudinally.

Figure 49-5. Blunt dissection is then used to develop the plane between the undersurface of the lateral gastrocnemius and the soleus muscles. The lesser saphenous vein and sural nerve are preserved and excluded from the flap. After developing this submuscular plane distally for several centimeters, and separating the lateral head from the medial head of the gastrocnemius in the posterior midline, the anterior and posterior incisions are deepened into the submuscular plane overlying the soleus muscle. The distal skin incisions must not extend farther than 10 cm proximal to the lateral malleolus, since the skin distal to this point is not acceptable as a random extension of this flap.

Figure 49-6. The distal transverse incision is made to a depth that preserves the areolar tissue over the Achilles tendon, yielding an acceptable bed for skin graft coverage. The distal dissection is carried in the subcutaneous plane until the caudal ending of the lateral gastrocnemius muscle belly is seen. The triceps surae tendon is then incised transversely at this point, and the plane of the proximal dissection continued deep to the gastrocnemius, but superficial to the soleus. The skin of the flap overlying the muscle is tacked with several sutures to the underlying muscular fascia, to prevent avulsion of the perforating vessels during dissection. These sutures are removed when the flap is inset into the defect.

Figure 49-7. Elevation of the myocutaneous flap is then continued until adequate rotation without tension is achieved to cover the defect. The proximal incisions can be developed to completely surround the vascular pedicle, creating an island flap, if needed for a greater arc of rotation. This maneuver is usually required only for defects that extend proximal to the knee.

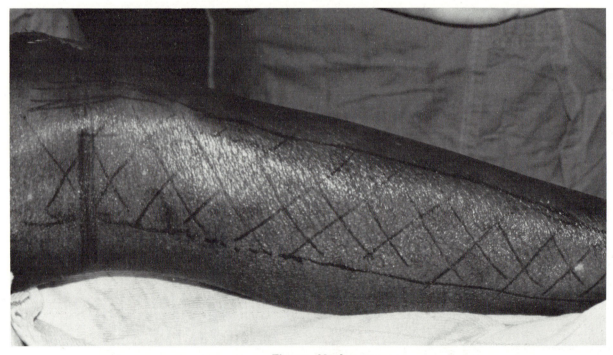

Figure 49-4

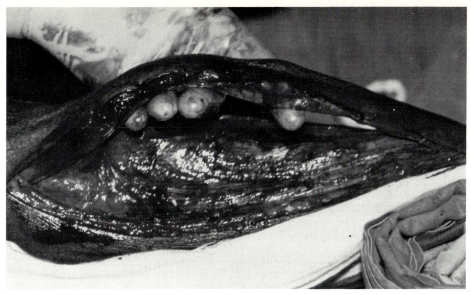
Figure 49–5

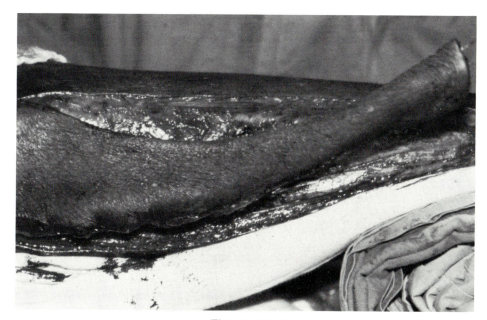
Figure 49–6

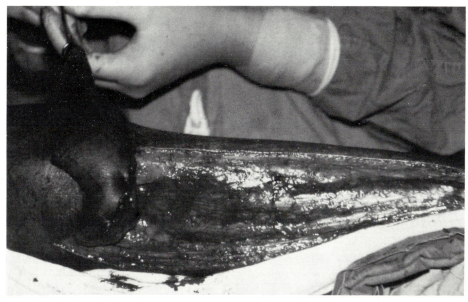
Figure 49–7

Figure 49–8. The flap is then transposed and sutured without tension, using interrupted or horizontal mattress sutures tied over large, soft bolsters to reduce and distribute pressure over the perimeter of the flap. The use of intravenous fluorescein has been recommended by McGraw to assess the circulation to the flap. After releasing the tourniquet one or two vials of fluorescein (500 to 1,000 mg) are injected intravenously, and after 20 minutes the surface of the flap is examined under ultraviolet light. The fluorescence should be intense and homogeneous over all portions of the flap. If the intensity is low, an additional dose of one or two vials may be given. Patchiness of fluorescence indicates interference with the vascular pedicle due to torsion or kinking, and must be rectified by repositioning the flap, or releasing soft tissue bands to insure flap survival.

The donor site on the calf cannot be closed primarily by suture, so that skin grafts are taken from the ipsilateral or contralateral upper thigh or buttock areas to resurface the donor defect. The calf wounds and skin grafts are dressed with supportive, occlusive dressings, with nonadherent medicated gauze placed over the flap suture lines at the knee. A posterior splint constructed of heat-labile material in the operating room is used to stabilize the knee and lower leg in the immediate recovery period. The splint must not encroach upon the base of the myocutaneous flap, or it would cause pressure on the vascular pedicle.

After a period of seven to ten days the skin grafts and other suture lines will have healed adequately to allow ambulation with supervision. The lower leg wounds may be supported with occlusive dressings or stockings, to avoid edema. If there is a need for secondary surgery to the knee joint or its supporting structures, this type of wound coverage provides a safe operative field that is durable and well vascularized.

Figure 49–9. Six weeks later, the portion of the lateral gastrocnemius myocutaneous flap overlying normal calf skin was transected and replaced into the upper lateral calf. By three months, excellent healing of the flap tissues resurfacing the anterolateral aspect of the knee is seen.

Pitfalls and Solutions

1. Proximal exposure of the two heads of the gastrocnemius muscle and identification of the soleus fascia must be done first. The medial and lateral heads of the muscle are separated prior to a distal dissection and elevation of the flap. Failure to take this initial step may result in injury to the vascular pedicle or in the flap being raised in the improper fascial plane.

2. As the dissection and elevation of the flap progress from distally to proximally, failure to temporarily suture the overlying skin to the gastrocnemius muscular fascia may result in disruption of the nutrient vessels to the skin of this flap, leading to necrosis.

3. Extension of the skin area at the distal margin of this flap farther than 10 cm proximal to the lateral malleolus will result in necrosis of the skin in that area. It is possible to delay this portion initially, transferring the lateral gastrocnemius myocutaneous flap with the distal skin extension at a later, secondary procedure. This length is not required, however, for defects in the immediate region of the knee.

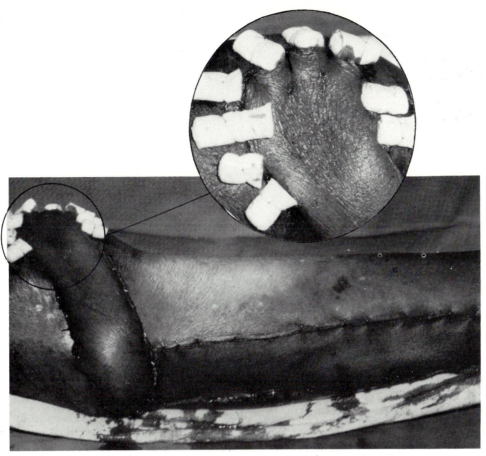

Figure 49–8

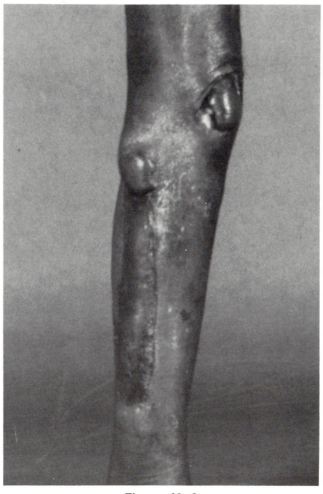

Figure 49–9

50

Knee: The Medial Gastrocnemius Myocutaneous Flap

The Problem

A deep burn of the anterior portion of the knee is a difficult problem because skin graft coverage is rarely stable over a long period of time. Local skin flaps are vascularized by random blood vessels, are often chronically scarred, and cannot be made of adequate surface area because of marginal blood supply. The medial gastrocnemius myocutaneous flap provides an excellent complement to the lateral gastrocnemius myocutaneous flap previously described for anterior, lateral defects.

Figure 50–1. This patient sustained a deep thermal burn occupying most of the anterior surface of the knee. The patella lay immediately beneath the granulating wound surface.

Technique

Figure 50–2. The medial head of the bicipital gastrocnemius muscle and its overlying skin receives a consistent arterial blood supply from the medial sural artery, which is a direct branch of the popliteal artery. The arterial pedicle courses from the popliteal artery for 2 to 5 cm before it enters the deep surface of the medial head of the gastrocnemius muscle. Two or three accompanying veins drain blood from this muscle into the popliteal vein. A branch of the tibial nerve runs with the vascular pedicle to innervate the muscle. The vessels enter the muscle and run axially for its entire length. No other arterial supply enters the muscle distally. Small-caliber myocutaneous vessels leave the superficial surface of the muscle, and anastomose in the subdermal plexuses of the skin territory overlying the muscle.

Figure 50–3. A pneumatic tourniquet is used to create a bloodless field. The contralateral upper thigh or buttock is used for skin graft donor sites, and is draped in the sterile field. The myocutaneous flap is outlined, with its anterior margin paralleling the medial edge of the tibia. The posterior margin is the posterior midline of the calf. The muscle ends quite consistently 4 to 5 cm distal to one-half of the distance between the popliteal crease and the ankle. A transverse incision is made distally, and the flap is raised in the bloodless plane between the medial gastrocnemius and soleus muscles, after the upper portion of the incision is made. Through the upper incision, the sural nerve and lesser saphenous vein are preserved whenever possible, and excluded from the flap. In the posterior midline a fascial layer is encountered, which is opened longitudinally to expose the juncture of the medial and lateral heads of the gastrocnemius.

Blunt dissection separates the two heads until the bloodless plane above the soleus muscle is reached. The entire medial head of the gastrocnemius muscle can then be elevated, using blunt dissection. The anterior and distal portion of the upper incision is deepened to this fascial level, and the distal portion may be extended to overlie the Achilles tendon if greater length is desired. This portion then becomes a random arterial extension of the myocutaneous flap. Preservation of the fine perforating vessels to the skin of the flap is insured by tacking the skin to the muscle fascia around the perimeter of the flap as it is being elevated. As the dissection of the distal skin portion of the flap proceeds proximally in a subcutaneous plane, the distal part of the gastrocnemius muscle is seen. At this point the triceps surae tendon is cut transversely, and the plane of flap elevation changes to the level previously developed overlying the soleus muscle.

KNEE: THE MEDIAL GASTROCNEMIUS MYOCUTANEOUS FLAP

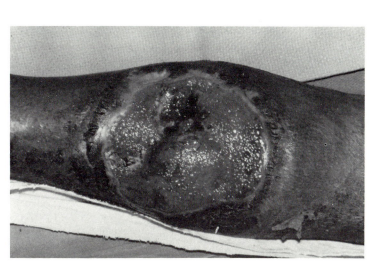

Figure 50-1

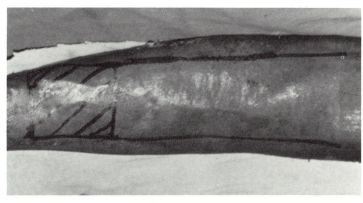

Figure 50-3

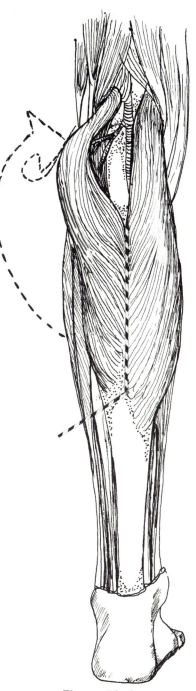

Figure 50-2

Figure 50–4. Rotation of the entire flap is easily accomplished, since the proximal vascular pedicle enters the muscle near the level of the knee joint. It is also possible to incise the proximal periphery of skin, through the subcutaneous tissue, and create an island pedicle flap, enhancing the capability of full rotation of the flap to areas even above the knee onto the distal thigh. The resulting flap is then sutured into place by means of half-buried, nonabsorbable mattress sutures. These sutures are tied over soft bolsters made of dental roll material, and spaced so as to distribute any tension over a wide area.

Figure 50–5. Split-thickness (0.014- to 0.018-inch) skin grafts are usually taken from the contralateral upper thigh or buttock to resurface the calf donor site. Suction catheters may be used beneath the flap after release of the tourniquet and achievement of hemostasis. As recommended by McGraw, one or two vials (500 to 1,000 mg) of fluorescein may be given intravenously to assess the vascularity of the transposed myocutaneous flap. This material will enter the circulation of the flap and diffuse, so that its presence can be visualized using an ultraviolet lamp. Twenty minutes must pass after intravenous injection to allow adequate diffusion of the substance. The fluorescence must be uniform in distribution and intensity when viewed with the ultraviolet light. Patchiness or low intensity may indicate kinking or torsion of the arterial pedicle. If the intensity of the fluorescence is uniform, but low, an additional intravenous dose of one or two vials (500 to 1,000 mg) of fluorescein may be given, and reassessment of the circulation in the myocutaneous flap carried out using the ultraviolet light.

Dressings and splints are applied as outlined for the lateral gastrocnemius myocutaneous flap.

Figure 50–6. This patient is shown six months after the initial operation. Two months before, the proximal portion of the flap was incised and returned to its original location at the medial calf. The surface of the knee is covered with well vascularized tissue that withstands the motions of the knee.

Pitfalls and Solutions

1. The work of McGraw, Mathes, Vasconez, and May should be consulted for the details of anatomy and flap design in various circumstances.

2. Attempts to develop this flap from distal to proximal without first exposing the two heads of the gastrocnemius muscle, and separation of the medial from the lateral portion and from the soleus fascia, may result in injury to the arteriovenous pedicle.

3. Suture of the muscular fascia to the overlying skin as the dissection proceeds will prevent avulsion of the skin and subcutaneous tissue from the muscle, with disruption of the perforating myocutaneous vessels.

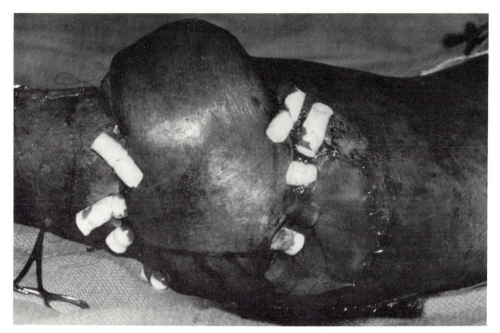

Figure 50-4

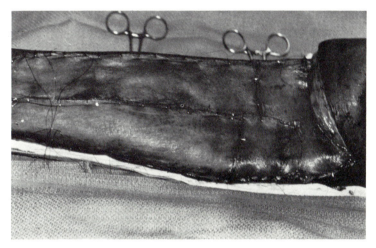

Figure 50-5

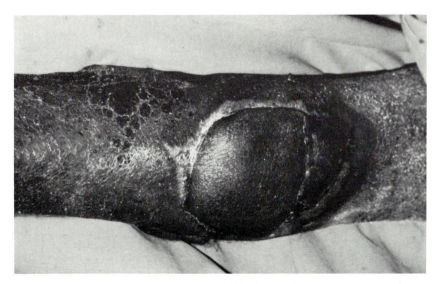

Figure 50-6

51

Coverage Near the Knee: The Sartorius Muscle Flap

The Problem

The potential occurrence of carcinoma in chronically unhealed burn scars must always be considered when assessing a patient for reconstruction.

Figure 51-1. A patient is shown in whom the burn injury many years before involved only the upper part of the leg and region of the knee. A medially-based cutaneous flap had been attempted previously, but failed because of inadequate length and surface area.

Figure 51-2. Chronic, recurrent ulceration developed distal to the knee. Thin, unstable epithelium was surrounded by scar in an area subject to tension during motion of the knee. The patient wanted no further scar placed upon the calf, since she could cover the proximal scars with a normal hemline. Thus, a reconstruction using distal tissue, such as a myocutaneous flap from the calf, was not feasible in this case.

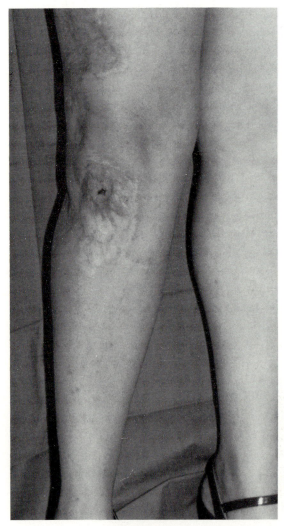

Figure 51-1

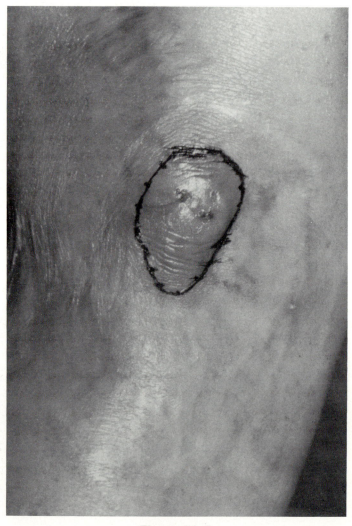

Figure 51-2

Technique

Muscle flaps for coverage of defects of the extremities and other parts of the body have been used for several years, and were popularized by Ger.

Figure 51–3. The sartorius muscle receives a dual blood supply: at its proximal and distal regions. The dominant vascular pedicle, however, is at the proximal portion of the muscle, consisting of branches of the lateral circumflex femoral artery and vein. The distal portion of the muscle is supplied by three or four arterial and venous branches from the distal femoral artery and vein. This distal blood supply is inconsistent to the overlying skin, and therefore makes a myocutaneous flap taken from the distal part of the muscle unpredictable. The central portion of the muscle is supplied by extensions of the proximal and distal vascular pedicles coursing through the muscle itself, with no direct branches of the femoral vascular system entering this area.

Figure 51–4. The chronically unhealed wound and surrounding scar is excised, and through a long, medial thigh incision the sartorius muscle is exposed. The muscle is divided across its upper central portion after extrafascial separation from the surrounding musculature.

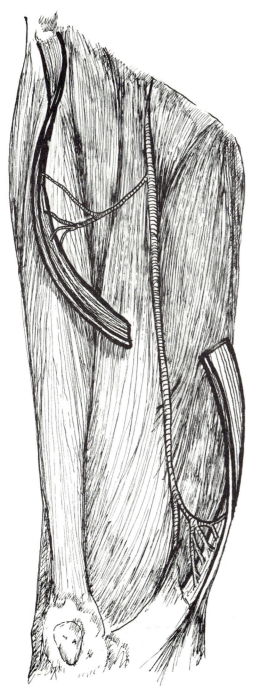

Figure 51–3

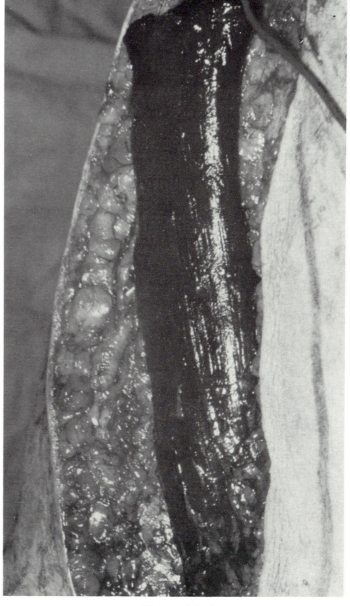

Figure 51–4

Figure 51-5. Sufficient length must be obtained so that the muscle may be turned backward and distally upon itself, and tunneled subcutaneously to the site of the knee wound. After the length of the distal sartorius muscle is tested, intravenous fluorescein is administered as described previously. The muscle should initially be placed in its anatomical position for this observation, and if intense, evenly distributed fluorescence is noted, the muscle is tunneled to its new position and the distal portion re-examined for adequacy of circulation. Any unfluoresced areas are excised, and the position of the muscle is readjusted.

The subcutaneous tunnel must be large enough so that undue pressure is not applied to the sartorius muscle or vascular pedicle as it passes through the tunnel.

Figure 51-6. After the muscle is positioned in the distal wound, it is tacked into place with several 4-0 synthetic, absorbable sutures. Medium-thickness, split-thickness skin grafts (0.014 to 0.018 inches) are taken and sutured into place with interrupted monofilament sutures. No external occlusive dressing is used, to avoid pressure on the transposed muscle in the wound, or over its subcutaneous course across the knee. A molded, heat-labile splint is made in the operating room, and applied to the leg with the knee in extension. Initial bulkiness of the muscle with overlying skin graft will be noted for several days. The patient is allowed to ambulate 10 to 12 days after surgery, wearing a posterior splint to prevent flexion of the knee for an additional three weeks.

Figure 51-7. Several months postoperatively there is durable skin cover, adequate contour, and no additional scar on the calf distal to the excised and resurfaced wound at the knee.

Pitfalls and Solutions

1. The length of muscle must be adequate for transposition, and is divided in its upper central portion. The circulation is tested while the muscle is *in situ* after division at this level, and after it has been transposed.

2. The subcutaneous tunnel must be large so that no pressure is applied to the vascular supply to the sartorius muscle at its base, or along the course of the tunnel over the knee.

3. Shearing forces causing graft necrosis, and edema leading to pressure necrosis of the transposed muscle, must be avoided. Therefore, flexion and extension of the knee is disallowed for three to four weeks postoperatively.

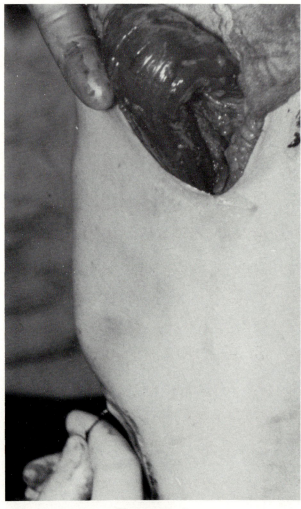

Figure 51-5

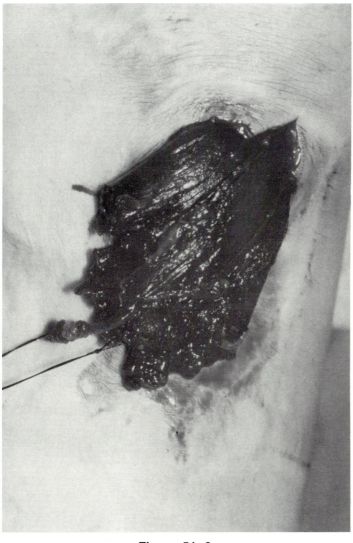

Figure 51-6

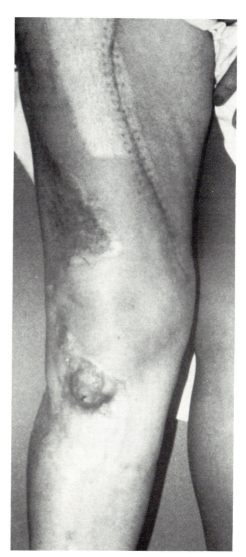

Figure 51-7

Foot: Plantar Surface Injury

The Problem

Deep thermal injury to the plantar surface of the foot is very unusual. Perhaps the commonest deep burn injury to this area is caused by either electricity (contact or exit wounds) or irradiation, such as ill-advised treatment for plantar warts. In the case of electrical contact or exit wounds, excision and split-thickness skin graft coverage frequently suffices. These grafts, when applied to adequately excised and prepared recipient sites, mature into durable, stable tissue coverage. Rarely, local, or possibly more distant, composite pedicle flap coverages of these wounds are required.

Technique

Figure 52–1. Irradiation injury to the plantar surface of the foot has produced a chronically unstable, progressively atrophic, and finally ulcerative wound not amendable to grafting. There is osteoradionecrosis of underlying metatarsal bone.

Figure 52–2. Since the distal toe is not involved, local pedicle flap coverage is easily accomplished by filleting it.

The chronic wound is completely excised, and the procedure includes resection of any underlying, osteonecrotic metatarsal head and/or shaft. A plantar incision is made that extends from the distal edge of the wound excision along the plantar midline of the toe. The neurovascular supply to the toe lies at the volar, lateral margins. Through the midline incision, the flexor tendons are identified and divided from their insertions on the phalanges. The toe is then filleted subperiosteally, which prevents injury to the neurovascular pedicles. In this manner the proximal two phalanges are exarticulated. At this point the distal midline incision is extended in a circular fashion around the distal toe, proximal to the nail bed, and the distal phalanx and nail area are excised. The filleted toe is then retracted proximally, and placed over the excision wound on the plantar surface of the foot. The metatarsal head has been resected, and its distal end is rounded and smoothed. The toe flap is then sutured into the recipient wound with 5-0 monofilament sutures, and a small drain is brought out through its proximal margin. An occlusive dressing is applied and the leg is elevated.

FOOT: PLANTAR SURFACE INJURY

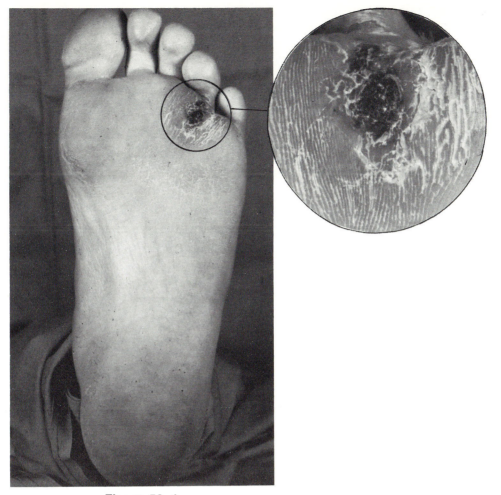

Figure 52-1

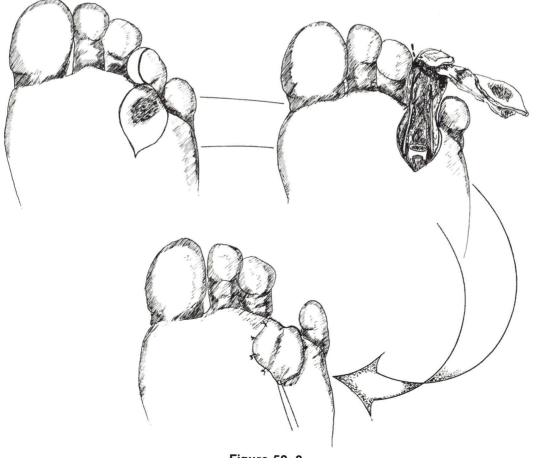

Figure 52-2

251

Figure 52-3. The healed flap is in position. This type of local pedicle flap will retain protective sensibility, and has excellent arterial and venous supply. Since the pressure points on the plantar surface of the foot are normally at the first and fifth metatarsal heads, and over the calcaneus, these more central, locally resurfaced wounds are protected from significant injury in the course of normal gait. Whereas a simpler split-thickness skin graft technique may be adequate for more superficial wounds, these local pedicles are required for deep injuries induced by irradiation or electricity.

Figure 52-4. The normal and reconstructed feet are seen while bearing weight, indicating the safety and low risk of using locally based pedicles when possible for distal plantar wounds. When these occur proximal to the central toes, shoe size, weight-bearing surfaces, and gait are unaffected.

Pitfalls and Solutions

1. Injury to the neurovascular pedicles to the filleted toe will result in necrosis. This must be prevented by cautious filleting of the toe from the midline, and bone resection is best done subperiosteally.

2. Any residual, exposed metatarsal present after resection must be reshaped to avoid pressure on the flap, which would lead to partial or complete necrosis of the flap when the patient ambulated.

FOOT: PLANTAR SURFACE INJURY

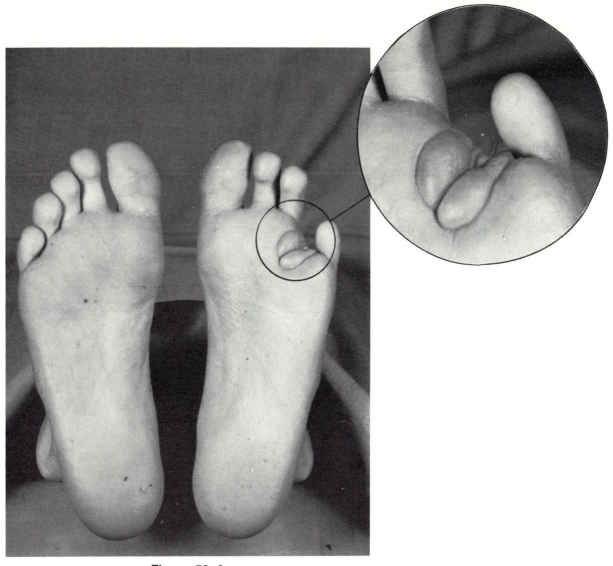

Figure 52–3

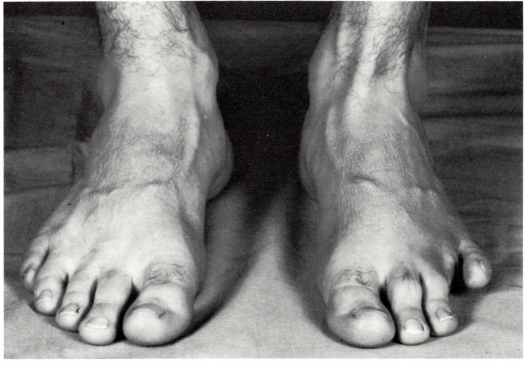

Figure 52–4

53

Dorsal Foot Contracture with Deformity of the Toes

The Problem

Adequate reconstruction of the dorsum of the foot after thermal injury requires the achievement of two goals: (a) durable, flexible skin coverage; and (b) restoration of the position of the toes for gait and shoe-fitting.

Since the normal, soft-tissue cover of the dorsum of the foot is relatively thin, as in the hand, an injury will often involve deep structures such as paratenon or tendon. The effect of this injury frequently is hyperextension of the proximal joints of the toes, with flexion of the distal joints, or "hammer toe" deformity. In many cases, debridement of the tendons is required because of direct injury, whereas in others, these structures become entrapped and foreshortened in a contracting dorsal foot scar. The "hammer toe" deformity is accentuated when the patient walks, because the fixed distal toe strikes early or coincident with the metatarsal heads, further causing the metatarsophalangeal joints to hyperextend. A marked range of flexion of the metatarsophalangeal joints is not required for a normal gait, but stable positioning of these joints, at least in a neutral attitude, is desirable for growth and the fitting of shoes. It is therefore crucial to carry out two important maneuvers when reconstructing the contracted dorsum of the foot:

a. Complete incision or excision of scar is necessary, including deeper structures when these are destroyed or foreshortened.

b. The toes must be not only repositioned in extension, but maintained in that position for several weeks during healing.

Less than adequate excision of scarred structures will leave secondary wounds that usually recontract after resurfacing. If the toes are not replaced at least into a neutral attitude, the wound for resurfacing will cover too small an area, and the "hammer toe" deformity will recur.

Technique

Figures 53–1, 53–2, 53–3. These typical deformities result from a burn scar of the dorsum of the foot. Malposition of the toes is marked, and it is clear that they will be pushed into further hyperextension during gait. The hypertrophic, foreshortened, soft-tissue cover of the dorsum will ulcerate repeatedly from friction in an ill-fitting shoe. Frequently the patient will have inadequate shoe-fitting because of unequal-sized feet, and the foreshortened foot will slide in its shoe.

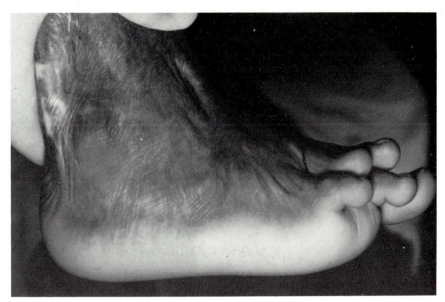

Figure 53-1

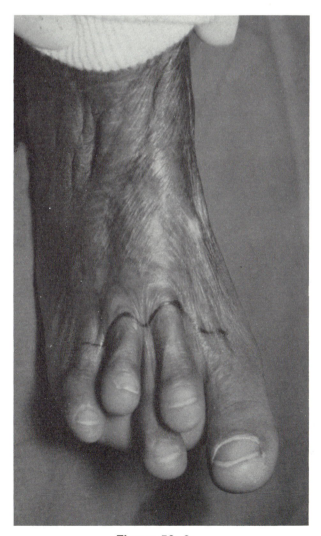

Figure 53-2

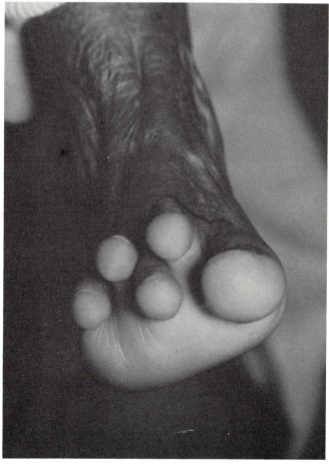

Figure 53-3

Figures 53–4, 53–5. A transverse incision is used, and any necessary undermining provided proximally and distally to allow extension of the toes. Any intact dorsal veins are preserved to minimize edema of the toes. If required, proximal and distal portions of the hypertrophic scar are excised until normal toe position is achieved, and if necessary, extensor tendons are divided or excised (not needed in the case illustrated).

Figure 53–6. It is then mandatory to maintain toe extension by means of interosseous Kirschner wires, crossing all the joints of the four toes. Thus, the wound is of maximal surface area, and is covered with a medium-thickness skin graft (0.014 to 0.018 inches). The interosseous wires are kept in place for six to eight weeks. If hemostasis is not perfect at the time of initial excision, the wound is dressed with the interosseous pins in place, and skin is grafted 24 to 48 hours later. An occlusive pressure dressing with nonadherent gauze directly over the skin graft is utilized, and the leg elevated for five to seven days. Weight-bearing and ambulation may be begun two weeks following surgery, and continued in a soft shoe or moccasin once the pins are removed and graft healing is complete. If edema is noted, a fitted pressure stocking is worn for several weeks after ambulation is begun.

Figures 53–7, 53–8, 53–9. Nine years after reconstruction of the foot, the patient demonstrated reasonable growth and contour, and was able to wear normal shoes.

Pitfalls and Solutions

1. Inadequate incision and excision will not produce a true maximum of wound surface area, and will cause a recurrence of the contracture.

2. Failure to maintain an extended position of the toes will cause recurrence of "hammer toe" and gait problems.

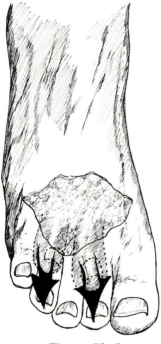

Figure 53–4

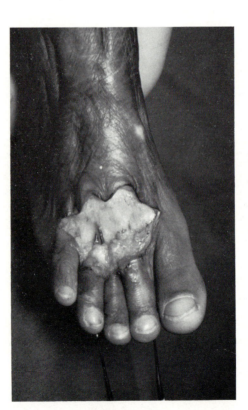

Figure 53–5

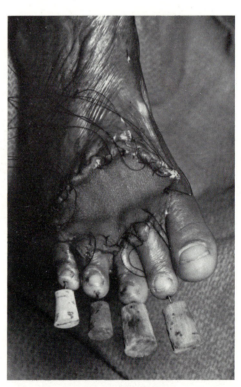

Figure 53–6

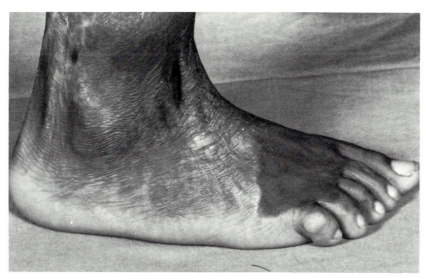

Figure 53-7

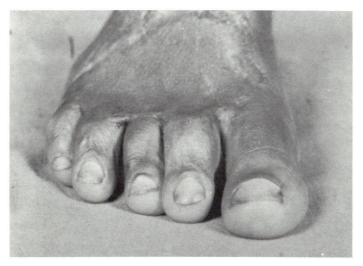

Figure 53-8

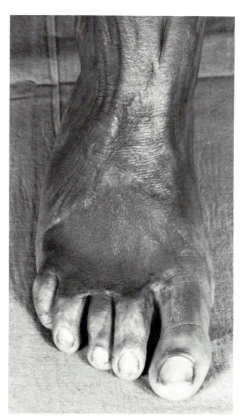

Figure 53-9

Cosmetics:
A Nonsurgical
Alternative

54
Cosmetics: A Nonsurgical Alternative

Regardless of his experience, knowledge, or technical virtuosity, the reconstructive surgeon is frequently thwarted by the scarred and discolored tissue that he must work with following thermal injury. Hypertrophic scar from healed second- and third-degree burns, or healed skin grafts over granulating muscle or bone, invariably limit the postoperative satisfaction of surgeon and patient. With the prospect of limited results, some patients (who often have had many surgical procedures) decline further reconstructive surgery. Artfully applied cosmetics may be of significant help to these patients, or to the one whom the surgeon believes he had nothing further to offer surgically. The main categories of deformity with which the cosmetologist may assist include:

a. Healed second-degree burns with color mismatch.
b. Depigmentation.
c. Hypertrophic raised scars.
d. Color mismatch of a skin-grafted surface without hypertrophic scar.
e. Partially destroyed or absent features.

The Problem

Figures 54–1, 54–2. This patient demonstrates hyperemic, healed second-degree burns of the right commissure of the mouth, check, and chin that draw the viewer's attention, nullifying the fact that she is actually very attractive. Because attention is focused on the lower third of the face, one also immediately notes the grafted neck. The goal of the cosmetologist in this case is to soften the color match and divert attention to the eyes, which are this patient's best facial features.

Technique

A heavy-coverage cosmetic base that adheres and looks natural is applied over only the scarred area, not the normal skin. The base is feathered onto normal skin until no line of demarcation exists.

A darker shade is then applied to anatomical points that are often in shadow — under the cheekbones, under the jaw, and the sides of the nose. This step tends to give the face a natural, balanced look.

A shade two to three tones lighter than the surrounding color is worked into the shadows under the eye and small, periobital expression wrinkles, to soften the tired or worried appearance.

Application of soft brown or black eye-liner to the inner and outer lash base area is followed by a soft, earth-colored shadow to the lashes, in keeping with the overall color of the patient. The most intense color is applied above the liner, fading as it approaches the brow area. A complementary color is applied below the base liner to prevent it from bleeding into the inferior eyelid area, as well as to intensify the eye color. Mascara is applied to the upper portion, tip, and lower portion of the lashes, in that order, taking care to avoid clumping. (A lash brush is helpful after mascara application.)

Rouge is applied, with the darkest color beginning below the zygomatic arch and blending down in a triangle to the base of the ear, to further dramatize the hollow of the cheek. The rouge is then lightened by mixing the base color, and applied above the hollow of the cheek, blending the two carefully and emphasizing or highlighting the "high cheekbones." Scarring is de-emphasized by using the base to cover the erythema and the skin, which has been contracted inferiorly.

Lip liner is used to redefine the outline of the lip. (The liner also helps to prevent bleeding of lip color into the fine vertical lines surrounding the lip, and intensifies the effect of the color.

An appropriate lip rouge (one pleasing to the patient) is carefully applied, preferably with a brush, which is more accurate and smoother, and gives a thinner, longer-lasting layer of color.

Powder is brushed on to "set" the make-up, allowed to stand ten minutes, brushed off, and then touched with a damp, fine-textured sponge to remove any excess.

This natural-looking make-up is now fully waterproof, and will last until removed with the proper cream.

COSMETICS: A NONSURGICAL ALTERNATIVE

The Problem

Figures 54–3, 54–4. Depigmentation is another common problem that is much more noticeable in dark-skinned people. This patient's face illustrates such a situation.

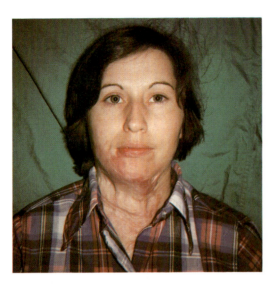

Figure 54–1

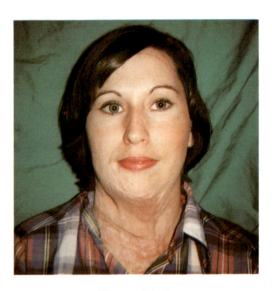

Figure 54–2

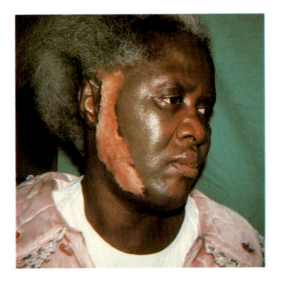

Figure 54–3

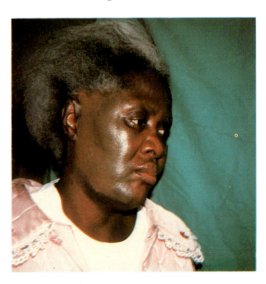

Figure 54–4

261

Technique

Color match can be improved by adding a brown shading cosmetic to the depigmented and black areas with a light, patting motion, feathering out the edges to blend with the prevailing surrounding skin tone. This blending should be done very carefully because it is a difficult coverage problem. The lighter skin tends to absorb color, and the cosmetic has to be reapplied at short intervals until set. When absorption ceases, the cosmetic is coated generously with powder, which is allowed to set for ten minutes, and then brushed off. The excess can be removed with a damp, fine-textured sponge.

The Problem

Figure 54–5. Hypertrophic, raised scars present a dimensional as well as a color problem. This child has large, hypertrophic scars in his nasolabial creases, which project above the normal planes of the face.

Technique

To minimize the visual effect, a light color is applied to match the surrounding normal skin, and particular care taken to apply the cosmetic thoroughly in the crevices of the scar. This color is mixed with a small amount of shade, and applied to the raised ridges, to soften them.

Figures 54–6, 54–7. Half of the face has been made up to reveal that the color can be softened and a good match obtained, but the improvement will still be only a modest one because of the projection of the scar from the face, as seen in the lateral view.

The Problem

Although a color mismatch of the face can often be avoided by taking skin grafts from above the clavicle, it is a frequent occurrence.

Figure 54–8. This patient, a 13-year-old male, has his hair pulled back to illustrate that all cosmetic facial units were grafted (with scalp skin). The result was a mixed one. Color match for the forehead, chin, and parts of the cheeks is excellent, but there is marked erythema and hypertrophic scar, especially in the nasolabial creases and over the zygomatic arches.

Technique

To achieve a smooth color match, the cosmetologist must know that shade and rouge have to be applied very sparingly to avoid a masklike or feminine look in the male.

The face is cleansed and a light skin-tone cosmetic applied to all affected areas, attempting to match the color of the unaffected visible skin. Shade is applied sparingly under the zygomatic arches, beneath the jaw, and along the sides of the nose. A blush of rouge is touched just over the zygoma. A light shade is applied to the grafted skin in the areas above and below the eye, to de-emphasize the supraorbital prominence and color difference.

Figures 54–9, 54–10. With half of the face made up, it is obvious that a color match with the surrounding normal skin can be achieved. The final effect, with the hair in a Prince Valiant cut, provides a soft frame for the face. The color of the face is lightened, and the youthful, bright eyes appropriately become the focal point.

Absent or partially destroyed features can be concealed by hair style as well as by cosmetics. For instance, this patient was missing the superior helix of the ear. The ear has a very low priority in reconstruction because it can be so easily concealed with the appropriate haircut, as accomplished with this Prince Valiant style.

The Problem

Figures 54–11, 54–12. This patient had a scalp graft performed to reconstruct his burned left eyebrow. Although there was a good surgical result, the hair growth was slightly thinner than on the normal side. It becomes quite noticeable because the color of the scarred skin around the eye draws attention.

Technique

An eyebrow pencil of the appropriate color is chosen. Shaping and density of the left eyebrow to match that of the normal right eyebrow is easily achieved. Medium shading is then applied to all the discolored skin around the eye and the nose, carefully working it into normal skin to blend naturally, with no line of demarcation. Darker shading is used to match the shadows seen on the normal side of the face, thus achieving color balance. Light shading is applied above and below the eye. It is quickly absorbed, and is reapplied several times until absorption stops. The result is natural and balanced, concealing the burn scars effectively.

In conclusion, the cosmetologist working with the burn team can offer solutions to some problems that are not amenable to surgical correction. Although everyone realizes that the patient will never regain his preburn appearance, our goal is a more limited one. We strive to give hope, to produce a reasonable appearance, and to offer the patient the opportunity to compete in work or school without fear of ridicule or embarrassment.

COSMETICS: A NONSURGICAL ALTERNATIVE

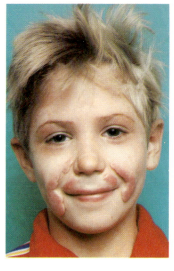
Figure 54-5

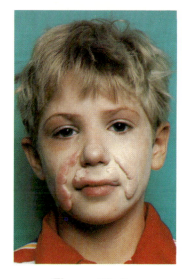
Figure 54-6

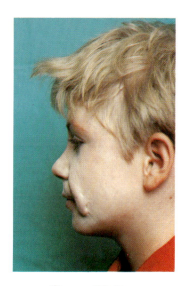
Figure 54-7

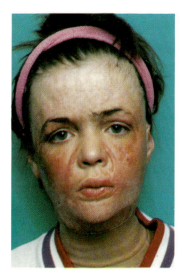
Figure 54-8

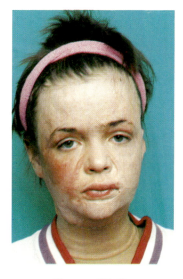
Figure 54-9

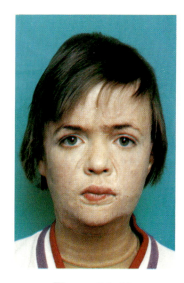
Figure 54-10

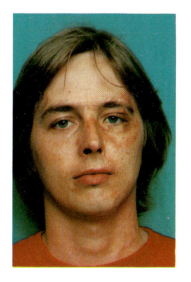
Figure 54-11

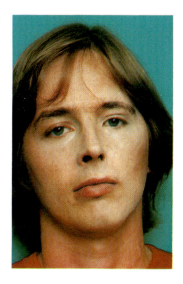
Figure 54-12

Index

Page numbers in *italics* indicate illustrations.

Abduction contracture, of small finger, 190–193, *191–193*
Accessory hand, 140–143, *140–143*
Adduction contracture, of thumb, 168–171, *168–171*
Advancement flap(s), in contracture of elbow, 112, 114, *112, 115*
  in reconstruction of axilla, 110, *110, 111*
  in thumb web, 172–173, *172–173*
Alopecia, burn, 4–7, *5, 7*
Amputation, selective, of fingers, 140–143, *140–143*
Areola, reconstruction of, 208–215, *209–211, 213–215*
Arthrodesis, for boutonnière deformity, 164
  interphalangeal, 160–163, *161, 163*
Axilla, reconstruction of, 108–110, *109–111*

Boutonnière deformity, 140, 156–163, 164–167, *141, 157, 159, 161, 164–167*
Breast, caudal displacement of, 196–200, *197, 199, 201*
  contracture of, 196–205, *197, 199, 201–205*
  diminished volume of, 206–211, *207–211*
  flap reconstruction of, 216–221, *217, 219, 221*
  lateral contracture of, 202–205, *202–205*

Capsulotomy, metacarpophalangeal, 156–159, *157, 159*
Cartilage, superior helix, loss of, 28, *29*
Cervical contracture, above hyoid, 90–94, *90–94*
  below hyoid, 102–105, *103–105*
  of anterior neck, 95–100, *95–101*
Chest. See *Breast*.
Chin, reconstruction of, 80–83, *80–83*
Compression mask, in reconstruction of lower face, 86, *87*
Contracture, abduction, of small finger, 190–193, *191–193*
  adduction, of thumb, 168–171, *168–171*
  dorsal adduction, of fingers, 186–189, *186–189*
  Dupuytren's, 144–148, *145–148*
  of axilla, 108–111, *109–111*
  of breast, 196–205, *197, 199, 201–205*
  of dorsal foot, 254–257, *255–257*
  of ear lobule, 30, *30, 31*
  of elbow, 112–115, *112–115*
  of fingers, 140–155, *140–143, 145–149, 151–155*
  of knee, 232–235, *232, 233, 235*
  of neck, 89–104, *90–99, 101, 103*
  of palm, 150–155, *151–155*
  of thumb, 134–136, *135, 137*
  of wrist, 132–137, *132, 133, 135, 137*
Cosmetics, 260–263, *261, 263*

Decortication, 22, *23*
Depigmentation, cosmetics for, 260–263, *261, 263*
Dermabrasion, in resurfacing of nose, 52, *53*
Digits. See *Finger, Thumb*.

Distant flaps, in contracture of elbow, 112
Dupuytren's contracture, 144–148, *145–148*

Ear, reconstruction of, 25–30, *26, 27, 29–31*. See also *Helix, Lobule*.
Elbow, contractures of, 112–115, *112–115*
Electrical injury, peripheral nerve loss from, 116–125, *117–125*
Esthetics, in reconstruction of face, 34–38, *34–37, 39*
Excision, of dorsum of hand, 144–149, *145–149*
Extensor tendon, of finger, in boutonnière deformity, 164–167, *164–167*
Eyebrow, cosmetics for, 262, *263*
  replacement of, 40–44, *41–44*
Eyelid, lower, reconstruction of, 50, *51*
  upper, reconstruction of, 46–49, *46, 47, 49*

Face, lower, reconstruction of, 84, 86, *85, 87*
Finger, arthrodesis of, 160–163, *161, 163*
  capsulotomy of, 156–159, *157, 159*
  contracture of, 144–149, 150–155, *145–149, 151–155*
    dorsal adduction, 186–189, *186–189*
  extensor tendon of, reconstruction of, 164–167, *164–167*
  hyperextension deformity of, 156–163, *157, 159, 161*
  pollicization of, 174–179, *174–179*
  small, abduction contracture of, 190–193, *191–193*
  syndactyly of, 180–185, *181–183, 185*
Flap, advancement, in axilla, 110, *110, 111*
  in thumb web, 172–173, *172–173*
  in upper lip, 55–57, *55–57*
  in amputation of finger, 140–143, *141–143*
  in burn syndactyly, 180–185, *181–183, 185*
  in contracture of elbow, 112
  in contracture of knee, 232–235, *233, 235*
  in face, 33
  in oral commissures, 62, *63*
  in superior helix, 26, *26, 27*
  myocutaneous, for anterior knee, 242–245, *243, 245*
    for ulcerated knee, 236–241, *237–239, 241*
    in breast, 216–221, *217, 219, 221*
    in groin, 228–231, *229–231*
  pedicle, in eyebrow replacement, 40, 42, *41, 42*
    in helix, 28, *29*
    in neck, 89
    in peripheral nerve loss, 124, *124, 125*
    in toe removal, 250–253, *251, 253*
    of scalp, 8–13, 22, *9–11, 13, 23*
  sartorius muscle, for knee, 246–249, *246–249*
  visor, of scalp, 14–17, *15–17*
  Z-plasty, in reconstruction of ear lobule, 30, *31*
Flexion deformity, of elbow, 112–114, *112–115*
Foot, 250–257, *251, 253, 255–257*
  contracture of, 254–257, *255–257*
  plantar surface injury of, 250–253, *251, 253*

265

INDEX

Genitalia, reconstruction of, 222–227, *222, 223, 225–227*
Graft, in adduction contracture of thumb, 171, *171*
   in caudal displacement of breast, 198–200, *199, 201*
   in contracture of elbow, 112–114, *112–114*
   in contracture of finger, 140–143, *140–143*
   in dorsal adduction contractures of fingers, 187–189, *187–189*
   in dorsal foot contracture, 256, *256, 257*
   in everted lower lip, 76–78, *76, 77*
   in lateral contracture of breast, 204, 205, *204, 205*
   in perioral reconstruction, 66–69, *67, 69*
   in peripheral nerve loss, 122, *122, 123*
   in pollicization, 178, *179*
   of anterior neck, 92–105, *92–99, 101*
   of axilla, 108–110, *109, 110*
   of eyelid, 50, *51*
   of face, 34, 38, *35, 39*
   of flap donor site, 240, 244, *241, 245*
   of genitalia, 224–227, *225–227*
   of hand, 139, 144–149, *139, 145–149*
   of interdigital web, 184, *185*
   of lower face, 86, *87*
   of lower labial sulcus, 74, *75*
   of lower lip–chin, 80, 82, *80, 81*
   of nipple-areola complex, 208–215, *209–211, 213–215*
   of nose, 54, *54*
   of palm, 150–155, *151–155*
   of scalp, 18–20, *19, 21*
   of upper eyelid, 46, *47, 49*
Groin, reconstruction of, 228–231, *229–231*

Hairline, restoration of, 14
Hammer toe, 254–257, *255–257*
Hand, 138–193. See also *Palm, Finger, Thumb, Syndactyly.*
   accessory, 140–143, *140–143*
   dorsum of, excision and grafting of, 144–149, *145–149*
   metacarpal, 138, 139, *138, 139*
Head, 3–87
Helix, reconstruction of, 25–29, *26, 27, 29*
Heterotopic ossification, 126–130, *126–130*
Hourglass procedure, 180–185, *181–183, 185*
Hyperextension deformity, of fingers, 156–163, *157, 159, 161*

Incision, of contracted palm, 150–155, *151–155*

Knee, contracture of, 232–235, *232, 233, 235*
   lateral, sartorius muscle flap for, 246–249, *246–249*
   resurfacing of, with myocutaneous flap, 242–245, *243, 245*
   ulcerated, 236–241, *237–239, 241*

Lip, lower, reconstruction of, 76–83, *76–79, 80–83*
   perioral hypertrophic burn scars of, 66–69, *67, 69*
   radiation injury of, 55–57, *55–57*
Lobule, ear, contracture of, 30, *30, 31*
   deformity of, 25

Mammoplasty, augmentation, 206–211, *207–211*
Mask, compression, in reconstruction of lower face, 86, *87*
Metacarpal hand, 138, 139, *138, 139*
Moulage, in reconstruction of lower labial sulcus, 72, 74, *73, 75*

Mouth, 55–78
   commissures of, reconstruction of, 58–64, *58–65*

Neck, contractures of, 89–104, *90–99, 101, 103*
Nerve graft, in peripheral nerve loss, 118, *118, 119*
Neurolysis, in peripheral nerve loss, 120–122, *120, 121*
Neurovascular island transfer, 124, *124, 125*
Nipple, reconstruction of, 212–215, *213–215*
Nose, resurfacing of, 52, 54, *53, 54*

Oral commissures, reconstruction of, 58–64, *58, 59, 61–65*

Palm, contracture of, 150–155, *151–155*
Pedicle flap, in burn syndactyly, 180–185, *181–183, 185*
   in eyebrow replacement, 40, 42, *41, 42*
   in peripheral nerve loss, 124, *124, 125*
   in reconstruction of helix, 28, *29*
   in removal of toe, 250–253, *251, 253*
   of neck, 89
   of scalp, 8–13, 22, *9–11, 13, 23*
Penis, reconstruction of, 222–227, *222, 223, 225–227*
Pericranium, destruction of, 18–20, *19, 21*
Perioral reconstruction, 66, 68, *67, 69*
Pollicization, 174–179, *174–179*
Priorities, in reconstruction of face, 38

Radiation injury, of lip, 55, 56, *55–57*
Radioulnar synostosis, 126–130, *126–130*
Rotation flaps, of scalp, 8–13, 22, *9–11, 13, 23*

Scalp, 4–23
   pedicle flap of, 22, *23*
   rotation flaps of, 8–13, *9–11, 13*
   visor flap of, 14–17, *15–17*
Scars, hypertrophic, cosmetics for, 262, *263*
Scrotum, reconstruction of, 222–227, *222, 223, 225–227*
Skin graft. See *Graft.*
Skull, loss of, 22, *23*
Splint(s), in abduction deformity of thumb, 134–136, *137*
   in adduction contracture of thumb, 171, *171*
   in boutonnière deformity, 164, *164*
   in dorsal adduction contractures of fingers, 188, 189, *188, 189*
   in everted lower lip, 76, 78, *78, 79*
   in heterotopic ossification, 130
   in hyperextension deformity of fingers, 156
   in reconstruction of anterior neck, 92, 94, 96, 99, 100, 104, *97, 105*
   in reconstruction of lower face, 86, *87*
   in reconstruction of lower labial sulcus, 70–75, *71, 73, 75*
   in reconstruction of lower lip–chin, 82, *82*
   in reconstruction of oral commissures, 64, *64, 65*
   of wrist, 132, *132, 133*
Sulcus, lower labial, reconstruction of, 70–75, *71, 73, 75*
Syndactyly, burn, 180–185, *181–183, 185*

Tendon(s), extensor, in boutonnière deformity, 164–167, *164–167*
Thumb, abduction deformity of, 134–136, *135*
   adduction contracture of, 168–171, *168–171*
   pollicization to create, 174–179, *174–179*
   web skin of, scarring of, 172–173, *172–173*

Toe, hammer, 254–257, *255–257*
   removal of, 250–253, *251, 253*
Trunk, 196–221

Upper extremity, 108–193

Visor flap, of scalp, 14–17, *15–17*
V-Y advancement, in reconstruction of ear lobule, 30

Web, interdigital, reconstruction of, 180–185, *181–183, 185*
   of thumb, scarring of, 172–173, *172–173*
Web formation, in axilla, 108, 110, *109, 110*
Wrist, contracture of, 132–137, *132, 133, 135, 137*

Z-plasty, in contracture of knee, 232–235, *233, 235*
   in reconstruction of ear lobule, 30, *31*
   in reconstruction of neck, 89
   in reconstruction of oral commissures, 62, 86, *63*